Psychiatry

D0094180

LECTURE NOTES ON

Psychiatry

PAUL HARRISON

DM, MRC Psych
*Clinical Reader and Honorary Consultant Psychiatrist,
University of Oxford*

JOHN GEDDES

MD, MRC Psych
*Senior Research Fellow and Honorary Consultant Psychiatrist,
University of Oxford*

MICHAEL SHARPE

MRCP, MRC Psych
*Senior Lecturer and Honorary Consultant Psychiatrist,
University of Edinburgh*

Eighth edition

b

**Blackwell
Science**

© 1964, 1968, 1972, 1974, 1979, 1984, 1989, 1998 by
Blackwell Science Ltd
Editorial Offices:
Osney Mead, Oxford OX2 0EL
25 John Street, London WC1N 2BL
23 Ainslie Place, Edinburgh EH3 6AJ
350 Main Street, Malden
  MA 02148 5018, USA
54 University Street, Carlton
  Victoria 3053, Australia
10, rue Casimir Delavigne
  75006 Paris, France

Other Editorial Offices:
Blackwell Wissenschafts-Verlag GmbH
Kurfürstendamm 57
10707 Berlin, Germany

Blackwell Science KK
MG Kodenmacho Building
7–10 Kodenmacho Nihombashi
Chuo-ku, Tokyo 104, Japan

First published 1964
Reprinted 1966
Second Edition 1968
Reprinted 1970
Third Edition 1972
Fourth Edition 1974
Reprinted 1976
Fifth Edition 1979
Portuguese Edition 1980
Sixth Edition 1984
Seventh Edition 1989
Reprinted 1991, 1993
Eighth Edition 1998

Set by Excel Typesetters Co.,
  Hong Kong
Printed and bound in Great Britain by
  MPG Books Ltd, Bodmin, Cornwall

The Blackwell Science logo is a trade
mark of Blackwell Science Ltd,
registered at the United Kingdom
Trade Marks Registry

The right of the Authors to be
identified as the Authors of this Work
has been asserted in accordance
with the Copyright, Designs and
Patents Act 1988.

All rights reserved. No part of this
publication may be reproduced,
stored in a retrieval system, or
transmitted, in any form or by any
means, electronic, mechanical,
photocopying, recording or
otherwise, except as permitted by
the UK Copyright, Designs and
Patents Act 1988, without the prior
permission of the copyright owner.

A catalogue record for this title
is available from the British Library

ISBN 0–632–03677–X

Library of Congress
Cataloging-in-publication Data

Harrison, P. J. (Paul J.), 1960–
    Lecture notes on psychiatry /
Paul Harrison, John Geddes, Mike
Sharpe.—8th ed.
      p. cm.
    Rev. ed. of: Lecture notes on
psychiatry / James Willis, J.A. Marks.
7th ed. 1989.
    Includes bibliographical
references.
    ISBN 0–632–03677–X
    1. Psychiatry—Outlines, Syllabi,
etc. I. Willis, James H. (James
Herbert), 1928– Lecture notes
on psychiatry. II. Geddes, John,
MD. III. Sharpe, Michael. IV.
Title.
    [DNLM: 1. Psychiatry
handbooks.   WM 34 W734L
1998]
RC457.W5   1998
616.89—dc21
DNLM/DLC
for Library of Congress   97–42431
                                CIP

DISTRIBUTORS
  Marston Book Services Ltd
  PO Box 269
  Abingdon, Oxon OX14 4YN
  (Orders: Tel: 01235 465500
            Fax: 01235 465555)

USA
  Blackwell Science, Inc.
  Commerce Place
  350 Main Street
  Malden, MA 02148 5018
  (Orders: Tel: 800 759 6102
            781 388 8250
            Fax: 781 388 8255)

Canada
  Login Brothers Book Company
  324 Saulteaux Crescent
  Winnipeg, Manitoba R3J 3T2
  (Orders: Tel: 204 224-4068)

Australia
  Blackwell Science Pty Ltd
  54 University Street
  Carlton, Victoria 3053
  (Orders: Tel: 3 9347 0300
            Fax: 3 9347 5001)

For further information on
Blackwell Science, visit
our website:
www.blackwell-science.com

Contents

Preface

Four per cent of medical students end up as psychiatrists. This book is meant to be equally useful to the 96% who don't, since we believe that the knowledge, skills and attitudes learned in psychiatry are relevant to all doctors — and other health professionals. We have tried to make psychiatry logical and enjoyable, and naturally to ensure that you pass the end-of-course examination. With these objectives in mind the structure of the book has been designed from the bottom up.

Why, what and how (Chapters 1–5)
The most important issue is how to actually 'do' psychiatry. After showing why psychiatry is worth studying and how to start (Chapter 1), we then take a radical(ish) approach to psychiatric assessment (Chapters 2–4) and explain how to make a diagnosis, plan management and communicate information (Chapter 5).

Causes, treatments and services (Chapters 6–8)
The second part of the book outlines the causes (Chapter 6) and treatments (Chapter 7) of psychiatric disorders. When describing treatment we have tried to be evidence-based and, wherever possible, justify our recommendations. Chapter 8 covers the organization of psychiatric services including important (but sometimes maligned!) topics like multidisciplinary teams and community care.

Disorders and settings (Chapters 9–18)
The features of adult psychiatric disorders are described in Chapters 9–15, followed by child psychiatry (Chapter 16) and mental retardation (Chapter 17). Since many psychiatric problems are dealt with in general practice and general hospitals, we finish with a summary of psychiatry in non-psychiatric settings (Chapter 18).

We thank Michael Gelder for encouraging a no-nonsense approach to psychiatry. We are grateful to the many colleagues who have shared their expertise with us, especially Philip Cowen, Christopher Fairburn, Michael Hobbs, Rupert McShane, Marion Perkins, Philip Robson and Dermot Rowe. The sins of commission and omission are entirely ours. We dedicate the book to Sandra, Rosie and Charlotte; Jane; Liz, Joe and Anna.

PJH, JRG and MCS
November 1997

CHAPTER 1

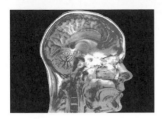

Psychiatry: Getting Started

Psychiatry can seem disconcertingly different from other medical specialties, especially if your first experience is on an inpatient unit. How do I approach a patient? What am I trying to achieve? Is he dangerous? Anyway, how do I tell if he's a patient or a member of staff? This chapter is meant to help orientate anyone facing the same situation. Like the rest of the book, it's based on three principles.

• Psychiatry is part of medicine.
• Psychiatric knowledge, skills and attitudes are relevant to all doctors.
• Psychiatry can be pragmatic, evidence-based, and no more 'waffly' than any other specialty.

1.1 What is psychiatry?

'Psychiatry is . . . mad, bearded men-in-white-coats in Gothic asylums using weird treatments on people who are untreatably mad or who are not really ill at all.' Though these cliches may once have had a grain of truth, the reality of modern psychiatry is very different. Psychiatry is fundamentally similar to the rest of medicine: it is based upon validated diagnostic and therapeutic principles which have success rates comparable to other specialties. Most of its patients are not 'mad' and are treated in the community. Psychiatrists don't wear white coats—and most don't have beards.

A better starting point is that *psychiatry deals with disorders of mental functioning — emotions,* *perceptions, thoughts and memories.* These disorders are often accompanied by motor and behavioural abnormalities (e.g. agitation, stereotyped movements) and somatic ones (e.g. loss of appetite, poor sleep). Their presence emphasizes that there is no distinction between mind and brain or between mental and physical: psychiatry is 'the medicine of the mind–brain', and its distinction from neurology is a matter of convenience and convention rather than anything more profound. Similarly, we prefer 'psychiatric disorder' to the older term 'mental disorder' since the latter can lead to misleading contrasts with 'physical disorder' and the implication that psychiatric disorders are somehow less real.

• Traces of this false dichotomy are still found in the use of the term 'organic' to refer to psychiatric disorders which have an identified pathological basis (Chapter 13).

1.1.1 Where's psychiatry going?

Psychiatry is in a phase of rapid evolution. Three contemporary themes permeate this book.

• *Psychiatry is becoming community-based.* Most psychiatric problems are seen and treated in primary care, with many others handled in the general hospital (Chapter 18). Only a minority are managed by specialist psychiatric services (Chapter 8). So psychiatry should be learned and practised in these other settings too — a point emphasized by the recent General Medical Council directives for the British medical student curriculum.

• *Psychiatry is becoming evidence-based.* Diagnostic, prognostic and therapeutic decisions should, of course, be based on the best available evidence. It may come as a surprise to discover that current psychiatric interventions are as evidence-based as they are in other specialties. Where possible we have indicated the strength of evidence for our treatment recommendations.

• *Psychiatry is becoming neuroscience-based.* Developments in brain imaging, molecular genetics and other areas are beginning to make real progress in the neurobiological understanding of psychiatric disorders. These developments are expanding the knowledge base and range of skills which the next generation of doctors will need.

1.2 Why study psychiatry?

The study of psychiatry is worthwhile for all trainee doctors, and other health practitioners, because the resulting *knowledge, skills* and *attitudes* are essential in every branch of medicine:

• a basic knowledge of specialist psychiatric disorders;
• a working knowledge of common psychiatric problems in all settings;
• the ability to assess someone with a 'psychiatric problem' effectively;
• skill in the assessment of psychological aspects of medical disorders; and
• a holistic approach to all patients.

1.2.1 Useful knowledge

Formerly, patients with severe psychiatric disorders were often institutionalized and their management was exclusively the domain of psychiatrists. The advent of community care (Chapter 8) has meant that other doctors, especially GPs, now encounter and participate in their management, so all doctors need basic information about these 'specialist' psychiatric disorders. They also need to be able to recognize and treat psychiatric problems, such as anxiety and depressive disorders, which are common in non-psychiatric settings and lead to significant morbidity (Chapter 18).

1.2.2 Useful skills

Most psychiatric disorders are diagnosed on the basis of the history, and many treatments are based on listening and talking. So, psychiatrists have had to retain particular expertise in: interviewing patients; assessing someone's mental state; and establishing a therapeutic doctor–patient relationship. Despite advances in biomedical science these skills remain important in all medical practice. For example:

• Making patients feel able to express their symptoms and feelings clearly, as a result of your empathy, interest, response to non-verbal cues, etc.

• Being able to use basic psychotherapeutic skills; for example, knowing how to help a distressed patient and how best to communicate bad news.

Without these 'soft' skills, the 'hard' skills of technological, evidence-based medicine cannot be fully effective. For example, an impatient, unempathic doctor is less likely to elicit symptoms needed to make a correct diagnosis, and a patient is less likely to adhere to the prescribed treatment if he distrusts or dislikes the doctor.

1.2.3 Useful attitudes

Psychiatric patients are still afflicted by prejudice and misunderstanding. You will see patients with severe symptoms in whom no cause or 'organic' pathology is found; their symptoms and disabilities are nevertheless real. You will be repeatedly reminded of the stigma which psychiatric patients experience from those around them. You will be confronted with psychological frailty. Recognizing these issues and dealing with them appropriately — developing positive, educated and effective attitudes — is another important aspect of studying psychiatry. Four 'good attitudes' are:

• recognition of the reality of suffering (and the possibilities for treatment) even when

there is no 'test' to prove it;
• awareness of the importance of psychosocial factors in all illnesses;
• awareness of the harm done by negative attitudes towards psychiatric disorder;
• acknowledging the role of your own personality in the doctor–patient relationship — your positive attributes as well as your vulnerabilities and prejudices.

1.3 How to start psychiatry

Now that we have briefly marked out what psychiatry is and the reasons for studying it, how do you start?

1.3.1 The psychiatric interview
The first, crucial, skill to learn is how to listen and talk (in that order) to patients: the *psychiatric interview*. This has two functions.
• It forms the main part of the *psychiatric assessment* by which diagnoses are made.
• It can be used therapeutically — in the psychotherapies, the communication between patient and therapist is the currency of treatment.

1.3.2 Psychiatric assessment
Because of its central importance, the principles of psychiatric assessment are outlined here. The practicalities are described in the next two chapters.

Psychiatric assessment has three *goals*:
• To elicit the information needed to make a diagnosis, since a diagnosis provides the best available framework for making clinical decisions. This may seem obvious, but it hasn't always been accepted in psychiatry.
• To understand the causes and context of the disorder.
• To form a therapeutic relationship with the patient.

Though these goals are the same in all of medicine, the *balance* of psychiatric assessment differs from other medical assessments.
• The interview provides a greater proportion of diagnostic information. Physical examination

and laboratory investigations only occasionally play a role.
• The interview includes a detailed examination of the patient's current thoughts, feelings, experiences and behaviour (the *mental state examination*') in addition to the standard questioning about the presenting complaint, past history, etc. (the *psychiatric history*').
• A greater wealth of background information about the person is collected (the *context*').

Psychiatric assessments have a reputation for being interminably long, a reputation which is only partly unfair. We take a pragmatic approach to the *process* of assessment. A *core assessment* is used to collect the essential diagnostic and contextual information (Chapter 2). Then, more detailed *modules* are used if anything has led you to hypothesize that the patient has a particular disorder (Chapter 3).
• This two-stage approach considerably shortens most interviews. It also happens to be what psychiatrists actually do as opposed to what they tell students to do!

1.3.3 Diagnostic categories
Solving a problem is always easier when you know the range of possible answers available. Similarly, before embarking on your first assessment, it helps to know the major psychiatric diagnoses and their cardinal features. Table 1.1 is a simplified guide. As experience is gained, aim for more specific diagnoses which correspond to those of the International Classification of Diseases, 10th revision (ICD-10) and which are used in this book.
• There is a widely used American alternative to ICD-10, called the Diagnostic and Statistical Manual of Mental Disorders (DSM-IV). The two systems are broadly similar.
• Whatever the classification, remember the underused category of 'no psychiatric disorder'.
• A term like *nervous breakdown* or *nervous trouble* has no psychiatric meaning — it may

Table 1.1 A basic guide to psychiatric classification.

Category	Example of disorders in the category	Basic characteristics	Common presentations
Organic disorder	Dementia, delirium	Impaired memory, 'organic' cause	Forgetfulness, confusion
Psychosis	Schizophrenia, bipolar disorder	Delusions, hallucinations	Bizarre ideas, odd behaviour
Neurosis	Anxiety disorders, hypochondriasis	Emotional disturbance	Worried, tired, physical complaints
Mood disorders	Depression	Low mood, loss of pleasure	Tearful, fed up, physical complaints
Substance misuse	Alcohol, opiate dependence	Psychological or physical effects of the substance	Addiction, withdrawal, depression
Personality disorder	Dissocial, paranoid	Dysfunctional personality traits	Exacerbation of traits when stressed
Mental retardation	Down's syndrome, autism	Congenitally low IQ	Developmental delay, physical features

describe almost any of the categories in Table 1.1.

Psychiatric classification

There are several principles and problems of psychiatric classification to be aware of:

• *Most diagnoses are defined by combinations of symptoms*, but some are based on aetiology or pathology. For example, depression can occur in someone with a brain tumour (diagnosis: organic mood disorder) or after bereavement (diagnosis: abnormal grief reaction), or without clear cause (diagnosis: depressive disorder). This combination of different sorts of category leads to some difficulties, which will become apparent later.

• *Comorbidity: many patients suffer from more than one psychiatric disorder* (or a psychiatric disorder and a physical disorder). So, if the diagnostic pieces don't seem to fit, there may be two jigsaws jumbled up in one box. The comorbid disorders may or may not be causally related, and may or may not both require treatment. As a rule, comorbidity complicates management and worsens prognosis.

• *Hierarchy: not all diagnoses carry equal weight.* Traditionally, organic disorder trumps everything (i.e. if it is present, coexisting disorders

are not diagnosed), and psychosis trumps neurosis. This principle is no longer applied consistently, partly because it is hard to reconcile with the frequency and clinical importance of comorbidity. Also, it is often unclear which is the primary category; a classic example is whether bipolar disorder (manic depression) is a mood disorder in which psychosis occurs, or a psychosis in which a mood disturbance occurs.

• *Psychiatric classification is not an exact science* and is open to several criticisms. Nevertheless, it does provide a degree of order upon which rational clinical practice can be based, by allowing diagnoses to be made which are reliable and useful for predicting treatment response and prognosis.

1.3.4 After the assessment: communicating information

Completion of the psychiatric assessment is followed by several steps:

• *Make a diagnosis*, whether definite, provisional or differential, using your knowledge of the key features of each psychiatric disorder.

• Attempt to understand how and why the disorder has arisen (Chapters 5 and 6).

• *Develop a management plan*, based on an awareness of the best available treatment (Chapter 7), on how psychiatric services are organized (Chapter 8), and on the patient's current circumstances, including their risk of harm to self or to others (Chapter 4).

• Communicate your understanding of the case and treatment plan (Chapter 5).

1.4 SUMMARY: KEY POINTS

• Psychiatry deals with disorders affecting emotions, perceptions, thoughts and memory. It also encompasses mental retardation, and the psychological aspects of the rest of medicine.

• Knowledge, skills and attitudes learned in psychiatry are relevant and valuable in all medical specialties.

• Be alert to the possibility of psychiatric disorder in all patients, and be able to recognize and elicit the key features.

• The major diagnostic categories are: neurosis, mood disorder, psychosis, organic disorder, substance misuse, personality disorder and mental retardation.

CHAPTER 2

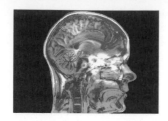

The Core Psychiatric Assessment

2.1 Approaches to psychiatric assessment

The psychiatric assessment as usually taught and described involves obtaining detailed, wide-ranging information about the patient (Table 2.1). This approach has the attraction that it is comprehensive and, once it is learned, it is easy to remember to ask about each topic. However, the disadvantages are considerable:

• Assessment can take an unrealistically long time.

• Information is collected irrespective of its clinical importance to the case. It may be difficult to tell the wood from the trees.

• It is hard to modify or abbreviate — one reason why psychiatric problems are neglected in medical practice.

We suggest a more flexible 'core and module' approach to assessment in which screening questions and other basic information (the core; see below) are used to identify possible diagnoses, which are then confirmed or excluded by more detailed assessment (the modules; Chapter 3).

• To use this strategy successfully you will need a working knowledge of psychiatric disorders and their symptoms in order to generate diagnostic hypotheses during the assessment. This stage of understanding will be attained rapidly — learning Table 1.1 and browsing through the key points at the end of each

chapter will give the basics. Until then, or if you feel unconfident, use the conventional assessment along the lines of Table 2.1.

Table 2.1 Headings for the complete psychiatric assessment.

Psychiatric history
Presenting complaint
Past psychiatric and medical history
Medication and other drugs
Family history
Personal history
Sexual history
Forensic history
Premorbid personality
Mental state examination (MSE)
Appearance and behaviour
Mood
Speech
Thoughts
Perceptions
Cognition
Insight
Physical examination

The mental state examination

The psychiatric assessment includes a mental state examination (MSE; p. 3) as well as the history. It's worth being clear about two aspects of the MSE which cause confusion:

• *What is the MSE time frame?* Formally, the MSE is limited to features apparent *during* the interview; everything else is history. In practice, the MSE is also used to assess *recent*

phenomena that have not been covered during the history (e.g. has the patient felt suicidal this morning?). Some examiners adhere to the division between history and MSE more rigidly than others.
• *Is the MSE the psychiatric equivalent of the physical examination in medicine?* To a degree it is — since it is where the '*signs*' of psychiatric disorder (i.e. observations made by the interviewer — 'patient keeps looking anxiously at ceiling') are elicited. However, the MSE also includes *symptoms* (experiences reported by the patient — 'I can hear an alien over there') and in this respect it overlaps with the functional enquiry (Fig. 2.1).

2.1.1 The 'core and module' psychiatric assessment

The *core* is a 'stripped-down' assessment designed to:
• obtain a clear account of the patient's main problem(s);
• screen rapidly but systematically for evidence of psychiatric disorder; and
• provide the background (contextual) information needed to guide immediate management.

The assessment then proceeds to one or more *modules* according to:
• the diagnostic suspicion(s) raised by the core assessment or other available information; and
• the need to exclude a disorder which, though unlikely, would be clinically significant.

The modules cover cognitive function, psychosis, mood disorder, neurosis, eating disorder, substance misuse and the unresponsive patient. Each is designed to confirm whether a disorder in that category is present and, if so, to establish the specific diagnosis. Each module also covers contextual information needed for the overall understanding of the case.

Assessment of childhood disorders, mental retardation and sexual functioning are covered in their respective chapters. Risk assessment is described in Chapter 4.

As an analogy for the core and module approach, consider a car journey from Oxford (presenting problem) to Edinburgh (diagnosis). The best route is that which allows the trip to be completed in the shortest time — something achieved by avoiding diversions and traffic jams. The conventional psychiatric assessment is like travelling along

Fig. 2.1 Venn diagrams comparing medical and psychiatric assessments, showing the relationship of history, functional enquiry, mental state examination (MSE) and physical examination. Note the overlap between the components of the psychiatric assessment. For example, recent suicidal thoughts might be detected in the history or MSE; akathisia (p. 63) may be elicited as a symptom in the history or MSE, or as a sign in the physical examination.

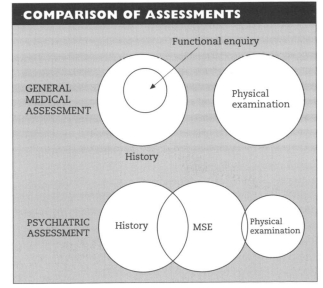

COMPARISON OF ASSESSMENTS

Functional enquiry

GENERAL MEDICAL ASSESSMENT

Physical examination

History

PSYCHIATRIC ASSESSMENT

History   MSE   Physical examination

predetermined (signposted) roads, regardless of traffic conditions — and stopping at all the sights recommended as 'worth a detour'. In contrast, in the core and module approach, the driver uses all the relevant information about traffic conditions to plan the route, and to modify it as conditions change on the way. He concentrates solely on reaching Edinburgh quickly and safely. He does not stop at sights en route (but notes their location as possible).

The way the interviewer moves from core to module, and the number of modules needed, will differ from case to case and will change as the interviewer gets more experienced (i.e. becomes better at generating good diagnostic hypotheses rapidly from the patient's clinical features). Three examples show how the assessment may develop.

A woman complains of tiredness. The core assessment reveals evidence of depression and a recent increase in alcohol intake, but not of suicidal intent, psychosis or cognitive impairment. You proceed to the mood and substance misuse modules which confirm the presence of a depressive disorder, but no significant alcohol problem.

A man is brought in having been found lying in the road screaming at passers-by to stop persecuting him. On this basis, you proceed to the psychosis and risk assessment modules regardless of what he may report during the core assessment (since he may initially deny symptoms in case you are part of the conspiracy). Given that illicit drugs can produce this kind of behaviour, you also use the substance misuse module.

A wife reports that her 70-year-old husband is getting confused. Your initial suspicions are of dementia, so you administer the cognitive module. However, though concentration is poor, he does not appear demented. Returning to the core, you find evidence of depression, so you move to the mood module which confirms that he has a severe depressive disorder (which in the elderly can present as apparent dementia).

If no modules have been triggered after completion of the core assessment and review of the case, it may be concluded that there is no evidence that the person has a psychiatric disorder.

2.2 Interviewing skills

Effective psychiatric assessment comes from knowing *what* questions to ask *when*. However, it also requires knowing *how* to ask them — to extend our analogy, the driver must be able to drive as well as navigate. So, before proceeding to the content of the assessment, we outline the skills which will increase your ability to get the necessary diagnostic information — and which ensure that the nature of the interview will help you develop a therapeutic relationship with the patient.

2.2.1 Before the interview
• Arrange the setting. Chairs are best placed at ninety degrees to each other. If a desk is required for making notes, this should not be directly between the patient and the interviewer.
• Try to arrange not to be interrupted.
• Read any referral letter and previous notes. These provide a preliminary diagnostic hypothesis, and may clarify the reason for the referral and suggest lines of questioning.

2.2.2 Beginning the interview
• Introduce yourself, check the identity of the patient, and make him comfortable.
• Sit in a relaxed and slightly forward posture.
• Describe the reason for the interview, the time available and the procedure to be followed.
• Emphasise confidentiality. If notes are to be taken, explain why.

2.2.3 Progress of the interview
• Begin by asking an open question such as 'How have you been feeling?'. Closed (but not leading) questions are used to clarify the

responses (e.g. 'Is it that you can't get to sleep or that you wake too early?').

• Encourage the patient to list the main problems and describe them in his own words.

• Keep control of the interview, yet allow the patient sufficient time to answer questions fully and in his own way. This balance can be the hardest skill to learn.

• Get answers that are as precise as possible— for example, estimates of symptom duration.

• As well as responding to what the patient says, be sensitive to non-verbal clues — for example, the patient's facial expression, posture or tone of voice.

2.2.4 Ending the interview

• Summarize your understanding of the case and ensure you've gained an accurate picture.

• Ask whether anything has been overlooked.

• Give an opportunity for the patient to ask questions.

• Explain what you plan to do next.

2.3 The core psychiatric assessment

The core psychiatric assessment covers the essence of the topics in Table 2.2 and is outlined below.

Table 2.2 The core psychiatric assessment.

Core history
  Reason for referral
  Presenting complaint(s) and their history
  Previous psychiatric and medical history
  Use of alcohol and drugs
Core mental state examination
  Appearance and behaviour
  Mood
  Speech
  Thoughts
  Perceptions
  Cognition
  Insight (attitude to illness)
Core contextual information
(Core physical examination)

• The accompanying notes provide background and rationale to the questions, plus a glossary of important terms.

2.3.1 The core history

Reason for referral
Who made the referral? Why?

> *Notes*
> • Clarify what questions the referrer wants addressed. This may give clues about the best way of approaching the interview and suggest initial diagnostic possibilities.
> • Identify the best informant available — someone to supplement and corroborate the history.

Presenting complaint(s) and their history
What does the patient think is the main problem?
Does the patient have any other problems? List them.
Assess the nature, duration and progression of the symptom(s).
Are there any precipitating and relieving factors? Has any treatment already been tried?
Assess degree of functional impairment: effect on relationships, work, sleep, etc.

> *Notes*
> • Getting a list of the patient's problems allows you to start generating diagnostic hypotheses. Some problems will be symptoms, others will represent the patient's predicament or provide the context of the disorder (e.g. homelessness).
> • The diagnostic importance of a particular psychiatric symptom is affected by its characteristics (intensity, fluctuation, etc.) and associated features. Knowing the relevant information to elicit comes rapidly with experience.

Psychiatric and medical history

Nature and frequency of any previous psychiatric contact, diagnosis and treatment.

Current medication and allergies?

Any serious medical illnesses or operations?

Notes

• About 50% of referrals have had prior psychiatric contact. A previous diagnosis is best seen as a strong hypothesis (i.e. it has a high pretest probability) to be tested. Past history may also provide useful information about prognosis and the patient's attitude to his disorder and its management.

• Psychiatric and medical disorders have many overlaps (Chapter 13); hence the need to elicit any significant past or current medical history.

Alcohol and drug use

How much does the patient drink in an average week?

If patient reports that he drinks alcohol regularly, ask the CAGE questions:

• Have you ever felt you ought to **C**ut down on your drinking?

• Have people **A**nnoyed you by criticizing your drinking?

• Have you ever felt **G**uilty about your drinking?

• Have you ever had a drink first thing in the morning (an '**E**ye-opener')?

Notes

• Alcohol and other substances may be a cause or consequence of, or an accompaniment to, psychiatric disorder. All are common, so substance misuse should always be briefly ascertained.

• The recommended limits for alcohol intake are 21 units per week for men and 14 for women (1 unit is half a pint of beer, a single measure of spirits or a small glass of wine).

• The CAGE is a useful screening tool. If three or more 'yes' answers are given, the likelihood ratio* for problem drinking is 250. If the patient answers 'no' to all four questions, the likelihood ratio is 0.2.

Repeat questions for any illicit drugs used.

2.3.2 The core mental state examination

The core MSE concentrates on aspects of the patient's recent mental state which are commonly affected by psychiatric disorder and which have diagnostic weight.

• Much of the core MSE will have been covered in the history, from observations made in passing or as part of a module already administered. However, the MSE is still useful to ensure that the presence or absence of all important recent phenomena are established and documented.

The headings of the core MSE are:

• *Appearance and behaviour* — much can be gleaned from careful observation of the patient's manner, movements and dress. An underestimated source of diagnostic information.

• *Mood* — disturbances of mood are very common. This section covers the main features of depression and the associated issue of suicidal risk.

• *Speech*—abnormal speech may be present in neurological, psychotic and mood disorders.

• *Thoughts* — thought content and the way thoughts flow are affected in many psychiatric disorders. The nature of the abnormality gives important diagnostic clues.

• *Perceptions* — mainly affected in psychotic and organic disorders.

• *Cognition* — cognitive impairment is characteristic of dementia and delirium. If severe, it may prevent a useful history from being taken.

---

* The likelihood ratio is the likelihood of a positive test result in someone who has the disorder/problem compared to someone who hasn't.

• *Insight* — lack of awareness of illness is classically a sign of psychosis or organic disorder, whilst the attitude to illness affects adherence to treatment and hence prognosis in all disorders.

Appearance and behaviour

Note the attitude of the patient to the interview and the rapport made.

Is the patient tearful, anxious, overactive or underactive?

Are there any unusual movements or eccentric behaviour?

Note the patient's physical appearance and dress.

Notes

• Psychiatric disorders are accompanied by characteristic changes in manner, emotional expression, physical appearance and movements. These often provide the first diagnostic clue. So, from the moment you meet, observe closely. For example, you may see:

— an ataxic man having problems getting to his chair. Could he have a frontal lobe tumour? Is he drunk?

— a patient avoiding eye contact and with little facial expression. He may be depressed.

— a tremor, suggesting Parkinson's disease or that she is taking antipsychotic drugs.

Mood

• Have you been low in spirits or depressed recently?

• Tell me how you've been feeling.

• Can you still enjoy the things that you normally do?

Ask about suicidal ideation. Use cues from the patient to broach the subject. For example:

• It sounds as if life's a bit of a struggle at the moment. Have you felt life isn't worth living?

• Would it be a relief if you didn't wake up in the morning?

• Have you actually thought of harming yourself in any way?

• Have you made any plans to end your life?

Notes

• Record both how the patient reports his mood (**subjective mood**) and also how it appears to you (**objective mood**).

• Always screen for mood disorders. They are common and some patients may not be aware of or do not complain of their mood symptoms.

• The best screening questions for depression determine the presence of persistent low mood and the loss of pleasure (**anhedonia**);

• Always assess suicidal intent. There is no evidence that asking about suicide increases the risk of it — the opposite is probably true.

• The mood section of the MSE can also reveal anxiety symptoms. Usually, however, these are detected more from the Appearance and Thoughts sections.

Speech

Does the patient speak spontaneously or only in response to questioning?

Is the patient's speech hard to understand? Is it because of articulation (dysarthria) or content (dysphasia)?

Notes

• Quiet speech which tails off or is monosyllabic is typical of depression; the opposite occurs in mania.

• Dysarthria suggests a neurological disorder or a side-effect of antipsychotic drugs.

• Dysphasia suggests a focal neurological disorder or thought disorder.

• Abnormalities in the content or flow of what is said are recorded in the next section.

Thoughts

Ask the patient to describe current preoccupations and worries.

- Do you have particular things on your mind at the moment?

Is the patient's train of thought difficult to follow? Try and describe how.

- Have you ever felt that people were against you?
- Have there been times when you felt that something strange was going on?
- Have your thoughts been directly interfered with by some outside force or person?

Notes

Abnormalities of thoughts and thought processes occur in many psychiatric disorders, and the precise form of the abnormality can be diagnostically important. Distinguish between the *content, nature* and *flow* of thoughts.

- *Thought content.* Record the presence and topic of predominant thoughts. For example:
  — recurrent worries about physical health in hypochondriasis;
  — a general theme of persecution in a paranoid psychosis;
  — a preoccupation with weight in an eating disorder.
- *The nature of the thoughts.* Regardless of its content, a thought may be normal or abnormal in nature. Three types of abnormal thought are recognized:
  — A **delusion** *is a false belief. It is firmly held despite contrary evidence and is out of keeping with the patient's cultural or religious background.* For example, a patient is absolutely convinced that he is the victim of an alien conspiracy (and so has locked himself in his flat and adopted a disguise). There may be one delusion or many, and they may be persistent or fleeting. Delusions carry special weight in the diagnosis of psychosis, so their recognition is an important skill. During the development and treatment

of psychosis, delusions may be partial, in that the patient realizes they might be false.
  — *An* **obsession** *is a recurrent thought, impulse or image that enters the subject's mind despite resistance.* The patient realizes that it originates from his own mind and may not be true, but he cannot resist thinking it and often has to act upon it (a compulsion). For example, obsessional thoughts about having dirty hands, the compulsion being to wash repeatedly. These symptoms characterize obsessive–compulsive disorder and also occur in depression.
  — *An* **overvalued idea** *is a belief not held quite as strongly as a delusion, and it is typically more 'understandable'.* It is typified by the belief of a girl with anorexia nervosa that she is fat.
- *The flow of thinking.* Even if the content of thoughts is normal, the flow (form) of thinking may not be. This is called thought disorder or *formal thought disorder.* It is often first detected if the patient is given time to reply at length to an open question, whereupon the interviewer realizes he is having problems following the train of thought. Write down a sample of what is said. Different sorts of thought disorder characterize schizophrenia and bipolar disorder.

Perceptions

Have you ever seen or heard things that other people couldn't?

Have you ever heard voices speaking when there was nobody there?

Do things or people seem different from normal?

Notes

- *A* **hallucination** *is a perception experienced as real in the absence of a stimulus.* For example, hearing a voice in the corner of the room when no-one's there. Hallucinations are pathognomonic of psychosis. They can occur in any modality; auditory ones are commonest. Like partial delusions, there are also partial hallucinations — usually called *pseudohallucinations* — which are perceived inside the head. They have little diagnostic significance. Similarly, hallucinations experienced whilst falling asleep (*hypnogogic*) or waking up (*hypnopompic*) are not abnormal.

• *An* **illusion** *is a misperception* — e.g. seeing someone in the shadows when there's no-one there. They have an 'as if' quality and in isolation have no diagnostic significance.

• **Depersonalization** *is a feeling of detachment from the normal sense of self —* 'as if I am acting'. **Derealization** *is similar, a feeling of detachment from the external world.* Both are a feature of neurosis but can be mistaken for the perplexity of psychosis.

Cognition

Is the patient orientated in time, person and place?

Is there clouding of consciousness?

Show the patient three items (e.g. watch, pen, shoe) and ensure they have registered them; test for recall 2 minutes later.

Notes
• Cognitive impairment is the hallmark of organic disorders — especially dementia and delirium. A lesser degree can occur in depression and schizophrenia.

• In delirium there is **clouding of consciousness** (usually manifested as decreased responsiveness to, or awareness of, surroundings); in dementia there isn't. See cognitive function and unresponsive patient modules.

• If the patient can recall the three items, the likelihood ratio for cognitive impairment is 0.06.

• If cognitive abnormalities are detected, physical examination and the cognitive function module are essential.

Insight

Do you think anything is wrong with you? If so, what?

Do you need any treatment? If so, what sort?

Notes
• Insight is a matter of degree, and fluctuates according to the mental state. It includes:

— the ability to recognize abnormal mental experiences as abnormal;

— appropriate recognition by the patient that he is suffering from a psychiatric disorder;

— acceptance of need for treatment.

• The patient's attitude affects management, especially the issue of compulsory admission.

2.3.3 Core contextual information

Recording of key details of the person's background and circumstances is part of the core assessment because they provide a *context* for the patient's problems. This helps in several ways:

• It enhances the therapeutic relationship by demonstrating an interest in the patient's problems.

• It identifies modifiable contributory problems (e.g. housing difficulties).

• It reveals personal factors which affect management (e.g. the presence of a supportive partner).

• It is necessary for understanding why the disorder has occurred.

• It sometimes helps diagnostically. For example, asking about employment reveals that a man lost his job for being late; further questioning shows this to have resulted from an unrecognized alcohol problem.

How much contextual enquiry is needed depends on the nature of the patient's problems, and what is already known. For example, in general practice the patient's circumstances will usually be well known; for an outpatient whose marriage and business are failing, extensive questioning would be needed to clarify the relationship of these problems to her depressive disorder.

Contextual information falls into three broad categories: *family history*, *personal history* and *current circumstances*.

Family history

Family tree, including grandparents, parents, siblings, children. Their ages, occupations, health.
Nature of the family relationships.
Family medical and psychiatric history.

Notes
• Problems in family relationships are commonly associated with psychiatric disorder.
• A positive family history is a risk factor for most psychiatric disorders.

Personal history

Childhood — health problems, school record.
Personality — the patient's usual attitudes, mood, beliefs, interests.
Relationship(s) — number, duration, type.
Employment history — nature of work, problems.
Criminal offences?

Notes
• Childhood problems can be associated with subsequent psychiatric disorder (e.g. conduct disorder with dissocial personality disorder).
• The premorbid personality shapes the risk, type and prognosis of psychiatric disorder. Ask simple questions about relationships, interests and prevailing mood. Offering alternatives may be helpful — e.g. 'Would you describe yourself as a loner or very sociable?'.
• A patient's view of their personality and life may be distorted during psychiatric disorder. For example, a depressed person will report themselves in an unduly negative light. *Always*

corroborate personality details from a close informant.
• The pattern of past relationships can give diagnostic clues, e.g. an absence of close relationships in schizoid personality disorder.
• The nature of employment gives clues to the patient's level of functioning. A deteriorating or disrupted work record may reflect a psychiatric disorder or a personality trait, respectively.
• Having a 'forensic history' (i.e. a criminal record) may be directly related to a psychiatric disorder or may be a coincidence. A history of violence will affect management regardless—see risk assessment (p. 36).

Current circumstances

Current relationships.
Current employment.
Current worries — finances, housing, relationship, etc.

Notes
• The current relationship is an important factor: it may have contributed to the disorder or have been damaged by it. Having a supportive partner improves outcome and assists management. Check the sex of the partner.
• All patients with severe psychiatric disorder are required to have an 'assessment of needs' (p. 80). Detailed information about the current circumstances is an essential component of this.
• Ongoing worries and stresses can perpetuate psychiatric disorder; their resolution is often part of management (e.g. sorting out a financial problem).

2.3.4 The core physical examination

The physical health of a psychiatric patient is important because:
• medical disorders can present with psychological symptoms. For example, lethargy and low mood may signify anaemia or carcinoma.
• patients with psychiatric disorders have

increased rates of medical illness, either because of a common aetiology or because the psychiatric disorder leads them to neglect their health.

So, in every assessment take account of the patient's physical appearance, and always consider what examination is required. This may include a brief examination of all systems. However, there is no prespecified physical examination in the psychiatric assessment since it depends upon the setting, the patient, the disorder and the treatment.

The setting. For example:

• A full examination is performed on every psychiatric admission because the psychiatrist takes medical responsibility whilst the patient is in hospital.

• In an emergency assessment, have a low threshold for examination since the possibility may not have been considered in the rush to refer the patient.

• In primary care, the GP may have examined the patient throroughly before referral.

The patient. For example:

• full examination if the patient has not been seen by a doctor recently;

• full examination if homeless, since at risk of tuberculosis, malnutrition, etc.;

• examine relevant systems if there is a history of a medical disorder.

The disorder and its treatment. For example:

• if alcohol misuse is suspected, examine for the physical signs which accompany it;

• patients on long-term antipsychotic drugs should be examined for tardive dyskinesia.

For patients receiving psychiatric care in the community, the responsibility for the patient's medical health should be agreed between psychiatrist and GP; usually it resides with the latter.

2.3.5 Core investigations

Core investigations in a medical sense do not exist in psychiatry, other than the convention that routine blood tests are performed on all psychiatric admissions. Elsewhere, investigations should be used to test a specific diagnostic hypothesis. For example:

• a urine drug screen in suspected drug-induced psychosis;

• extensive biochemical, imaging and genetic investigations in a 30 year old with dementia;

• a brain CT or MRI scan in someone with delirium and a history of a fall;

• thyroid function tests in a patient with anxiety, palpitations and weight loss;

• renal function and ECG in a patient you plan to start on lithium treatment.

2.3.6 Shrinking the core: a 'one-minute screen' for psychiatric disorder

The core assessment is portable for use in all settings, not just in specialist psychiatry. However, there are occasions when only a moment can be spent on psychiatric assessment. Even this is worthwhile. The following seven questions screen rapidly for the psychiatric disorders common in general practice or the general hospital. (Table 2.3)

• A positive response to any question should lead to a core and module assessment.

Table 2.3 Seven screening questions for psychiatric disorder.

Question	Screening for:
In the past month:	
1. Have you felt low in spirits?	*depression*
2. Do you enjoy things less than you usually do?	*depression*
3. Have you been feeling generally anxious?	*neurosis (anxiety)*
4. Are you worried about your health or other specific things?	*neurosis (health anxiety)*
5. Has your eating felt out of control?	*eating disorder*
6. Do you drink alcohol? If so, ask CAGE questions (p. 10)	*alcohol problem*
7. Present 3 items and ask patient to recall them after 2 minutes.	*dementia/delirium*

2.4 SUMMARY: KEY POINTS

- The aim of psychiatric assessment is to gather sufficient information to make a diagnosis and set it in context.
- Most information comes from the history and mental state examination. Physical examination and investigations play much lesser roles.
- Diagnostic hypotheses should be made and tested throughout the assessment.

- The flexible approach combines a core assessment with modules which are used when the likelihood of a specific diagnosis is raised.
- Psychiatric disorder can and should be rapidly screened for in all medical settings.
- Interviewing skills allow you to gather information efficiently.

CHAPTER 3

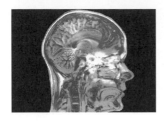

Psychiatric Assessment Modules

3.1 Using assessment modules

The purpose of the core assessment is to screen efficiently and rapidly for features associated with a high probability of the presence of a psychiatric disorder. The modules are used to confirm or refute these diagnostic hypotheses, as illustrated by the examples on p. 8.

• Each module contains general advice about areas to cover, plus suggestions for specific questions as well as explanatory notes and definitions of key terms.

• The clinical features of each disorder are also summarized in the relevant chapter. So, for example, the question 'Is this man depressed?' can be approached using the mood module and the mood disorders chapter (Chapter 9).

• There is no distinction between history and mental state examination in the modules.

• More than one module is often needed.

• Other types of assessment are covered elsewhere: risk (Chapter 4), sexual functioning (Chapter 11), children (Chapter 16) and mental retardation (Chapter 17).

We do not suggest reading this chapter in one go. Instead, read a module as you come across a clinical problem requiring its use.

3.2 Assessment of cognitive function

3.2.1 Using the cognitive function module

'Cognitive function' comprises attention, memory and language. It is the first module, since impairment in these areas interferes with the psychiatric assessment, sometimes to the point that no useful history can be gleaned from the patient.

Triggering the cognitive function module

The suspicion of cognitive impairment may have arisen for many reasons. For example:

• the patient has done poorly on the core cognitive screen;

• the patient is muddled, as judged by their manner or response to initial questions;

• there is a history of forgetfulness;

• there is a history of a medical disorder associated with cognitive impairment;

• the patient is old (e.g. at age 90, he has a 20% chance of dementia).

Differential diagnosis

Once the presence of cognitive impairment has been established, the main distinction is between *dementia* and *delirium*. Cognitive function can also be affected in depression and some neurological disorders, so evidence for these other causes of cognitive impairment is also sought.

Related modules

If the person can't or won't answer questions, use the *unresponsive patient* module. The *mood* module is often needed. Cognitive impairment can affect ability to self care, so *risk* assessment is necessary too. If there is long-standing impairment, consider *mental retardation* (Chapter 17).

3.2.2 The cognitive function module

The module is based around the *mini-mental state examination (MMSE)*, a validated screen of cognitive functioning which is widely used in clinical practice. (The MMSE is distinct from the mental state examination) If cognitive impairment is found, the module then aims to discover its cause.

• Before proceeding, read the cognition section of the core MSE (p. 13).

The mini-mental state examination

1 'What day of the week is it?' (Score 1)
2 'What is the date?' (1)
3 'And the month?' (1)
4 'And the year?' (1)
5 'What is the season?' (1)
6 'What country are we in?' (1)
7 'The county?' (1)
8 'The town [city/village]?' (1)
9 'The hospital or the street?' (1)
10 'The name of this ward?' [The name/number of this house?] (1)
11 Name three objects (e.g. clock, table, umbrella) and ask patient to repeat them. (Score 1 for each one recalled correctly after one presentation — max. 3.) If any failures, repeat names until all three registered.
12 'Spell "world" backwards.' (Score 1 for each letter in correct order; max. 5)
13 Point to a pencil and a watch and ask patient to name them. (2)
14 'Now could you tell me the three objects that I named a few minutes ago?' (3)

15 Ask patient to repeat 'No ifs, ands or buts'. (1)
16 Tell patient to carry out this task: 'Take this paper in your right hand, fold it in half, and put it on the floor.' (Score 1 for each part; max. 3)
17 Show the patient a piece of paper on which is written 'Close your eyes' and ask them to do what it says. (1)
18 Ask patient to write a short sentence of her choice. (Score 1 if it makes grammatical sense—ignore spelling)
19 Ask patient to copy this figure:

(Score 1 if both shapes are five-sided and the intersecting lines make a quadrangle)

Notes

• Normal score is 25–30. A score of 21–25 suggests dementia or delirium (likelihood ratio = 5); 20 or less is highly suggestive (likelihood ratio = 8).
• Ensure the patient has registered each question — don't be misled by hearing or visual problems or by lack of attention.
• Language impairment and apraxias occur in dementia as well as in focal neurological disorders.
• ***Confabulation*** (fabrication of recent events to cover gaps in memory) occurs in amnesic syndrome (p. 133).
• Unawareness of self identity is rare even in severe dementia, and raises the possibility of a dissociative disorder (p. 101).

Assessing the cause of cognitive impairment

Assess for features of delirium:
Is the person drowsy?
Are they fully aware of their surroundings?
Are they distractible? Irritable?
Are they hallucinating?

When did the problems start?
Administer the depression module.

Notes

• The hallmark of delirium is *clouding of consciousness*—drowsiness, distractibility, delusions and visual hallucinations. There is usually an acute onset and fluctuating course.
• Depression can also cause cognitive impairment.
• If neither delirium nor depression is present, the diagnosis is almost certainly dementia.

Other components of the module

Do a careful physical examination. Look for evidence of infection, vascular disease, thyroid status and alcohol abuse. The neurological examination should include testing of cranial nerves and evaluation of cortical functions (e.g. apraxias, hemineglect, primitive reflexes).

Obtain corroboration of the history (e.g. of duration and severity of the impairment) from an informant.

Notes

• If dementia is diagnosed, proceed to assess: (a) its likely cause; (b) its effect on daily living; and (c) any associated problems. These issues are covered in Chapter 13.
• Delirium is due to a variety of medical conditions, many of which need urgent treatment. Sometimes, dementia is reversible too. Thus, a medical history and physical examination followed by appropriate investigations are essential whenever cognitive impairment is found.
• Talk to the informant first if the impairment is severe — see also the unresponsive patient module.

3.3 Assessment of psychosis

3.3.1 Using the psychosis module

The aim of the module is to determine if psy-

chosis is present and, if so, whether it is schizophrenia or another psychotic disorder.

• The cardinal features of psychosis (delusions, hallucinations, lack of insight) were defined in the core assessment (p. 12).
• The diagnosis of schizophrenia relies on detailed evaluation of several symptoms and signs, so the module is quite long.

Triggering the psychosis module

Psychosis may be suspected for diverse reasons, such as:
• delusions elicited in the core assessment;
• bizarre or inexplicable behaviour;
• history of amphetamine use;
• being found in a neglected state, refusing help; or
• man heard talking and laughing to himself in a police cell.

Differential diagnosis

Once it is established that the patient is psychotic, the differential diagnosis is between:
• schizophrenia — *first-rank symptoms* (p. 22) play an important part in the diagnosis;
• psychosis in depression or mania;
• an organic or drug-induced psychosis; and
• psychosis not fitting into any of these categories (e.g. delusional disorder).

Related modules

Given this differential diagnosis, the module is usually accompanied by the *mood* and *substance misuse* modules. The *cognitive function* module may be indicated since concentration and memory can be impaired during psychosis. Risk assessment is needed as psychoses commonly lead to a risk of harm.

3.3.2 The psychosis module
Appearance and behaviour
Note manner and dress.

Notes

• *Manner*—patient may be suspicious (are you part of his delusional conspiracy theory?), distracted (is he hearing voices?)

or distant and uninterested (negative symptoms of schizophrenia (p. 115)).
• *Dress* — some people with schizophrenia dress idiosyncratically. For example, a man wore a silver foil hat to prevent his thoughts being extracted.

Movements
Is there abnormality of movements or posture?
Is the patient restless?
Are there mannerisms?

Notes
• Motor abnormalities occur in psychosis and, commonly, as side-effects of antipsychotic drugs.
• The side-effects include *dystonia, parkinsonism, akathisia* and *tardive dyskinesia* (p. 63).
• A **mannerism** is a regular, repetitive movement or gesture which is complex and seemingly purposeful. A repeated simple and purposeless one is a **stereotypy**. Both occur in schizophrenia.
• *Catatonia* describes a group of motor signs which are rare but characteristic of catatonic schizophrenia (p. 115):
— *echopraxia/echolalia* (the patient imitates the interviewer's every action/word)
— *automatic obedience* (compliance with all instructions regardless of consequence)
— *ambitendency* (tentative movements back and forth—as if unsure what to do)
— *posturing* (*catalepsy*) (the maintenance of inappropriate or bizarre postures)
— *waxy flexibility* (limbs held in externally imposed positions—muscle tone is increased)
— *negativism* (seemingly motiveless resistance to all instructions or attempts to be moved).

Mood
Does the overall mood seem normal? Is it responsive?

Is the emotional expression appropriate with the topic being discussed?

Notes
Psychosis can occur with depression or mania, hence use of mood module. Here, only the abnormalities of mood occurring in schizophrenia are mentioned.
• *Flattened affect* is a decrease in emotional responsivity and expression, even when emotionally charged topics are discussed. It is a negative symptom of schizophrenia. Distinguish from depression and parkinsonism.
• *Incongruous affect* is emotion not in keeping with the topic being talked about.

Speech
Are made-up words used or words used idiosyncratically?

Notes
• A **neologism** is a word invented by the subject, usually invested with a personal meaning. Be sure the patient doesn't just have a larger vocabulary than you!

Thoughts—content
Is there any evidence of delusions?
• Is anything bothering you at the moment?
• Do you believe or understand things differently from other people?
• Do people have a special interest in you? Are people against you? How do you know?
• Is anything on the TV referring to you particularly?
• When did you first realize this (i.e. the delusional belief) was true? How?

Notes
• Since, by definition, a delusion is believed to be true, its detection requires the interviewer to be receptive to clues and sometimes to 'go along' with implausible statements in order to elicit more details. For example, a man matter-of-factly asked one of us how we were affected by the Bulgarian mafia—the first hint of his psychosis. A non-committal

reply led him to elaborate and reveal his persecutory delusional system.

• Different sorts of delusions have been defined.

— A *delusional perception* is a delusional interpretation of a normal perception. For example, a man saw a woman sneeze and knew this meant he must leave town. It is sometimes preceded by a sense of unease or perplexity (*delusional mood*).

— In a *delusion of reference*, an event or message (often on TV) has a unique meaning for the person.

— A *secondary delusion* is one which arises understandably from another mental state abnormality (e.g. delusion of guilt in depression); a *primary delusion* doesn't.

— Delusions may be classified by content. The commonest are *persecutory* delusions, in which the person is the victim of perceived injustice or conspiracy. G*randiose* delusions are seen in mania, *nihilistic* ones in depression.

Thoughts — flow and possession

Is it difficult to follow the meaning of what the patient is saying? Write down a representative sample.

Do the person's thoughts seem to flow normally?

• Do your thoughts sometimes stop suddenly?

• Are your thoughts sometimes removed from your head?

Does the person feel in control of their thoughts and actions?

• Do your thoughts get put into your head from outside?

• Do you ever feel that other people can influence your thoughts or actions?

Are the thoughts experienced unusually?

• Are other people aware of your thoughts?

• Do any of your thoughts get repeated in your mind like an echo?

Notes

• In schizophrenia thought disorder, the connections between thoughts are obscure and there is a rambling quality. Descriptive terms include **knight's move thinking**, *loosening of associations* and *word salad*. For example: 'I got on the bus when I saw the man from the hostel, in the next street where I was. You know I've seen that dog again? Still, whatever time it was . . . '. A different type of thought disorder occurs in mania (p. 26).

• In schizophrenia abnormalities also occur in the perceived source, ownership and fate of thoughts:

— *Thought insertion*: thoughts are perceived to originate elsewhere and be put into the patient's head.

— *Thought withdrawal*: the experience of thoughts being removed from one's mind.

— *Thought broadcast*: the subject experiences his thoughts being available to and heard by others. Hearing one's own thoughts repeated is called *thought echo*.

— *Thought block*: the flow of thoughts abruptly ends. Distinguish from a simple loss of concentration, and from thought withdrawal.

— *Passivity*: thoughts, feelings or actions are experienced as being under external control. For example, a schizophrenic patient who killed her son described being unable to resist carrying out this act because of the 'force' controlling her.

Perceptions

Does the person seem to be hearing things which are not there?

• Do you hear voices when there doesn't seem to be anyone present?

• Can you describe them?

• What are they talking about?

• Do they talk directly to you or about you?

• Do they comment on what you're doing?

• Do they want you to harm yourself or other people?

Repeat similar questions for hallucinations in other modalities.

Notes
• The characteristic hallucinations of schizophrenia are *third person auditory hallucinations* (i.e. hearing the voice talking *about* you). Sometimes these take the form of a *running commentary* on the patient's actions.
• *Somatic hallucinations* (e.g. buzzing sensations due to a beehive implanted in the chest) and hallucinations in other modalities also occur. *Visual hallucinations* suggest an organic psychosis. *Olfactory hallucinations* and sensory distortions occur in temporal lobe epilepsy.

Cognition
Is the patient disorientated?

Notes
• An acutely psychotic patient may be distracted by his experiences and perform poorly on cognitive testing. Try and distinguish from delirium.
• Patients with chronic schizophrenia may underestimate their age by several years and show other signs of mild cognitive impairment.

Other components of the module
How does the patient explain their experiences/sensations?
• Do you think you are ill in any way? Do you need help?

Take a developmental history including complications of pregnancy or delivery.

Any family history of psychosis?

Any history of substance misuse?

Corroborate history with informant.

Perform physical examination, concentrating on neurological system.

Notes
• Insight is characteristically but variably impaired in psychosis. *Distorted awareness of reality* is a related term which conveys what is often apparent to the interviewer.
• Early developmental events and family history are risk factors for schizophrenia.
• Alcohol and illicit drugs can induce psychosis. Consider substance abuse module.
• Organic disorders can produce psychosis (Chapter 13), hence relevance of medical history and physical examination.

First-rank symptoms of schizophrenia
A number of symptoms in this module are *first-rank symptoms*, accorded great significance in the diagnosis of schizophrenia. They are summarized in Table 3.1.

Notes
• For definitions, see text.
• The likelihood ratio for schizophrenia is > 4 if a first-rank symptom is present. However, they are not pathognomonic — first-rank symptoms occur in other psychoses, and not all schizophrenics have had one.

Table 3.1 First-rank symptoms of schizophrenia.

Delusions
   Delusional perception
Hallucinations
   Thought echo (audible thoughts)
   Third person auditory hallucinations
   Running commentary
Thought flow and possession
   Thought withdrawal
   Thought insertion
   Thought broadcasting
Passivity
   Passivity of thought, feelings or actions

- They are sometimes called *Schneiderian* symptoms after the psychiatrist who described them.
- Listing first-rank symptoms is a favourite exam question.

3.4 Assessment of mood

3.4.1 Using the mood modules
There are separate modules for lowered mood (*depression*) and for elevated mood (*mania*).

Triggering the depression module
The module will be used frequently — depressive disorders are common, as are depressive symptoms in other diagnoses. Examples of the triggers for this module include:
- detection of a depressive symptom or suicidal thought in the core assessment ;
- unexplained fatigue;
- any of the presentations in Table 9.2, p. 85.

Triggering the mania module
The mania module may be triggered by:
- detection of manic symptoms in the core assessment;
- recent grandiose or disinhibited behaviour;
- a past history of bipolar disorder.

Related modules
Depression can overlap or coexist with so many other diagnoses that any of the other modules may well be necessary. The presence of mood disturbance requires risk assessment (mainly for suicide risk) as well.

3.4.2 The depression module
Appearance and behaviour
Does the patient look depressed? Is he crying? Is he agitated?
Is there good eye contact?
Is there a normal range of emotional expression?

Notes
- In depression there is often decreased eye contact and a lack of expression and movement — called *psychomotor retardation*. Other depressed people are *agitated*, pacing to and fro or wringing their hands.

Speech
Is the speech normal in speed, loudness and amount?

Notes
- In severe depression, speech is slow, quiet and sparse. Sentences tail off, as though the patient cannot summon the energy or concentration to continue.

Mood
Has the patient noticed a change in mood?
- How have you been feeling in your spirits?
If appropriate:
  - How long have you felt this way?
  - Do you still enjoy the things that you usually do?
  - Is your mood lower at a particular time of day?
  - Do you often feel like crying?
  - Do you easily get irritable?

Notes
- The duration, pervasiveness and severity of these symptoms affects diagnosis and management.
- *Anhedonia*, the lack of pleasure from normally enjoyed activities, is an important symptom of moderate and severe depression.
- *Reactivity of mood*: In severe depression, the normal reactivity of mood to circumstances is lost.
- *Diurnal variation of mood*: mood is worst early in the morning, improving as the day goes on.
- The predominant subjective feeling in depression may be sadness, irritability or lethargy.

Sleep, appetite and other bodily functions

- How are you sleeping at the moment? Do you have problems getting to sleep or waking early?
- What is your appetite like? Do you enjoy your food? Have you lost weight?
- Are you constipated? (How are your periods?)
- Has your interest in sex changed recently?

Notes

- Biological rhythms and drives are impaired in depression.
- Sleep is affected in several ways. *Initial insomnia* is common when there is accompanying anxiety. Sleep is shallow and unrefreshing. *Early morning waking* is the most characteristic change, often occurring with diurnal variation of mood, so the patient is awake and at his most desperate when the rest of the world is asleep.
- Appetite is reduced, resulting in weight loss and contributing to constipation.
- Irregular periods or amenorrhoea occur in women.
- There is a general loss of energy and libido.

Thoughts — content

- Do you see things getting better? What would improve things?
- How do you see yourself compared with other people?
- Do you feel guilty about anything you have done?
- Do you feel that you are of value?
- Do you have worries about your physical health?
- Do you feel that people are getting at you? If so, is it justified?

Ask in detail about suicidal thoughts (p. 38).

Notes

- Prevailing thoughts have a negative colouring, centring upon perceived failures, low self-esteem, and so on.
- Feelings of hopelessness and guilt are important as they lead to thoughts of suicide.
- The content of thoughts (and the person's appearance) may suggest accompanying anxiety—covered in the neurosis module.
- Worries about health and complaints of physical symptoms are common in depression.

Thoughts — nature

Are any of the thoughts obsessional in nature?
- Do you find yourself checking things repeatedly?
- Do you like things especially clean and tidy?
Are any of the thoughts delusional in nature?

Notes

- Obsessional thoughts are common in depression. If they are prominent, consider obsessive–compulsive disorder and use the neurosis module.
- Delusions are rare in depression as a whole, but characterize psychotic depression. They tend to be *mood congruent* (i.e. depressive in nature).

Perception

Are there hallucinations? What are they like?

Notes

- Hallucinations sometimes occur in psychotic depression — usually second person voices saying derogatory things.
- Depressed people may describe that sensations are less intense than usual and they feel isolated from the normal emotions and activities of the outside world.

Cognition

Is concentration impaired?

• What is your concentration like? Can you read a paper or follow a TV programme?

Is there objective evidence of cognitive impairment?

Notes

• Depression can produce cognitive impairment, called *pseudodementia*, contributed to by lack of motivation, concentration and self-confidence. It must be distinguished from dementia, as it responds to treatment of the depression.

Other components of the module

Does the patient think they are depressed?

Identify past and current stressors — marital strife, unemployment, etc.

How has the patient tried to cope with the problems?

Is there a past history of mood disorder? What has its course been? What treatment worked?

Does the person have depressive traits in their personality?

Is there a family history of psychiatric disorder or suicide?

Notes

• Severely depressed patients may deny that their mood is abnormal and decline treatment.

• Stressors (*life events*) can precipitate depression; identifying them helps make sense of the depression — and can be therapeutic.

• Coping strategies adopted by patients may lead to additional problems. For example, use of alcohol.

• Many patients with depression have had previous episode(s) of mood disorder. Ask about their nature, treatment and outcome.

• Depressive personality traits may affect the risk and outcome of depressive disorders. An informant should provide the personality information (p. 14).

• A positive family history is a risk factor for depressive disorder and suicide.

3.4.3 The mania module
Appearance and behaviour

Note manner and dress.

Is the patient distractible or irritable?

Notes

• Clothes and make-up may be bright and garish or dishevelled.

• Look out for flamboyant or disinhibited gestures. The patient may try and hug you, snatch your notes or challenge your qualifications.

• A manic person may be unable to concentrate enough to give useful answers. If so, focus on eliciting current symptoms and take the rest of the history later or from an informant.

• The predominant emotion can be euphoria and infectious gaiety, or sudden and extreme irritability.

Speech

Is the speech fast? Excessive in amount? Hard to interrupt?

Notes

• Speech in mania is fast, loud, expansive and hard to interrupt (*pressure of speech*). It reflects the underlying pressure of thoughts and the person's attempts to share their many wonderful ideas.

Mood

Has the patient noticed a change in mood recently?

• Do you feel happier than usual? More confident?

Notes

• Some people with mania deny their mood is elevated, or are too busy to think about it.

• Mood can be labile, or *mixed* — simultaneous depressive and manic features.

Sleep, appetite and other bodily functions

- How are you sleeping? More or less than usual?
- How is your appetite?
- Has your interest in sex changed?

Notes

- Tiredness and sleep drive are decreased. A manic patient may stay up all night working or playing.
- Appetite may be increased, or the patient may be too busy to eat.
- Libido tends to be enhanced and sexual activity uninhibited.

Thoughts — content

- What's on your mind at the moment?
- Do you have special powers or abilities?

Are these thoughts grandiose or implausible?

Notes

- Thoughts are expansive and grandiose. There may be a single, preoccupying scheme (e.g. to build a football stadium in the garden) but usually there is a kaleidoscope of incomplete, jumbled ideas.

Thoughts — nature

Are the thoughts delusional in nature?
Any evidence of unwise or dangerous ideas?

- Have you got plans to spend a lot of money?
- Can you do things which most people might find impossible?

Does the train of thought jump from one topic to another?

Notes

- In mania (but not the milder *hypomania*), the grandiose ideas become delusional. Religious themes are common — e.g. the patient knows he is the Messiah. Sometimes delusions are dangerous—e.g. the belief that one can drive excessively fast, or fly, or borrow unrealistic amounts of money. Take these

beliefs seriously—the unpredictability of mania means they may suddenly be acted upon.

- *Flight of ideas* is a type of thought disorder which occurs in mania. Thoughts shift rapidly from one thing to another, with understandable connections between them based on puns, rhymes and other associations. For example: 'I'm fine, a fine wine, whining and moaning like Jonah . . . Jonah Louis . . . pooeeee wooee. . . .' Write down a snippet.

Perception

Any evidence of hallucinations?

Notes

- Mood-congruent auditory and occasionally visual hallucinations occur. For example, the voices may tell the person what special powers they have or suggest ways in which they can save humanity.

Other components of the module

Does the patient think they are unwell or need treatment?
Corroborate recent history, especially with regard to unusual and inappropriate beliefs and actions.
Recent use of illicit drugs or alcohol?
Past history of mania or depression?
Has patient ever been prescribed lithium? Is he supposed to be taking it now?
Family history of mood disorder?
Perform a physical examination.

Notes

- Insight fluctuates in mania. A person may seem aware of their condition and the need for treatment one moment but not the next.
- An informant usually paints a more dramatic picture of recent behaviour than does the patient. Gather evidence of specific dangerous or out-of-the-ordinary behaviours, since they affect management,

e.g. whether patient should be detained, or needs a pregnancy test.
- Manic episodes can be caused by drugs, especially amphetamine, and sometimes by alcohol.
- Bipolar disorder is treated prophylactically with lithium, and sudden discontinuation can precipitate mania. Ask the patient if they take lithium; if unsure of compliance do a blood level (p. 61).
- Bipolar disorder is strongly familial.
- Physical examination is indicated since mania can be due to an organic disorder (e.g. frontal lobe tumour), especially if the first episode occurs in middle age or beyond.

3.5 Assessment of neurosis

3.5.1 Using the neurosis module

Neuroses are emotional disorders usually involving anxiety and manifesting as psychological or bodily complaints. They include anxiety disorders, stress reactions and somatoform disorder.
- Neurosis is a broad and complex category. It is correspondingly difficult to distil into a limited number of questions, and its assessment may take a while to get to grips with. We suggest you read Chapter 10 in conjunction with the module.

Triggering the neurosis module

Neurotic symptoms are extremely common and the neurosis module is easily triggered. For example:
- a man who looks tense or anxious
- a woman who is preoccupied or clearly worried about something
- someone distressed after a recent trauma
- a patient with bodily symptoms without apparent medical cause.

Related modules

Neurotic symptoms often coexist with depression, so the *depression module* will nearly always

be necessary. Use the *substance misuse* module if there is evidence of alcohol or drug use as a cause of, or response to, the symptoms. Worries about food or body image will trigger the *eating disorders* module.

3.5.2 The neurosis module
Appearance
Does the patient look tense, anxious or worried?

> *Notes*
> - Anxiety is a state of arousal and may be apparent from the person's appearance and behaviour.

Anxiety
Open questions:
- Have you been worrying a lot about things recently? What about?
- Do you feel wound up or tense?
- Do you suffer from aches and pains?
Characterizing the anxiety:
- Are the feelings there most of the time, or in specific situations? Such as?
- Do you get sudden 'attacks' of anxiety? How does your body feel then?
- Can you put your worries out of your mind?
- Do you avoid doing things because of your worries?

> *Notes*
> - Anxiety consists of *psychological* symptoms (e.g. tension, fear) and *bodily* symptoms (e.g. palpitations, sweating). Either can predominate.
> - Anxiety is usually *situational* (*phobic*), occurring in response to a specific stimulus. Less commonly it is *generalized* or *free floating*.
> - Anxiety can also be paroxysmal—a *panic attack*: a sudden, discrete episode of severe anxiety which builds rapidly then gradually subsides over about an hour.
> - People rapidly learn to avoid situations in which they feel anxious or uncomfortable. They may first present for

help because of the practical problems which avoidance produces.

Obsessions and compulsions

- Do you get recurrent unpleasant images or thoughts?
- Do you find that you have to keep checking things? Or keep things very clean and tidy?
- What do you do? How many times?
- Do you try to resist the thoughts or the urge to respond to them? If so, what happens?

Notes

- *Obsessions* and *compulsions* (p. 12) are characteristic of obsessive–compulsive disorder and also occur in depression and anankastic personality disorder.

Other symptoms

Enquire about medically unexplained symptoms:

- How is your health generally?
- Do you have medical problems your doctor can't explain?
- Do you worry you might have a serious disease?
- Do you suffer from severe tiredness or exhaustion?
- Have you ever lost your memory, sight or the use of part of your body?

Ask about major life events:

- Have you ever been in a major accident or trauma?
- How has it affected you?

Has the person felt detached or distant from themselves or their surroundings?

Notes

- Many people have unexplained somatic complaints such as pain or fatigue, or a belief that they have an undiagnosed disease. Often they have other symptoms of an anxiety disorder or depressive disorder; if not, consider *somatoform disorder*.
- Medically unexplained fatigue is the

main feature of *neurasthenia* (*chronic fatigue syndrome*). Fatigue and lethargy also occur in depression and anxiety disorders.

- *Dissociative disorders* are neuroses in which there is loss of function (e.g. amnesia, paralysis). They are usually encountered in medical settings (e.g. after admission for neurological investigation).
- Major trauma can lead to *post-traumatic stress disorder* (PTSD). Reliving of the trauma in flashbacks or nightmares is characteristic.
- Feelings of detachment from self or surroundings (*depersonalization–derealization*) are a common symptom of neurosis, may occur in healthy people when tired, and are occasionally a diagnosis in their own right. Such feelings are hard to describe (e.g. 'It's as if there's glass between me and the world') and must be distinguished from psychotic symptoms.

Other components of the module

When did the symptoms start? Did they seem related to recent events and stresses?

How has the person coped? Any treatment to date?

How do the symptoms interefere with the person's functioning?

Is the person a frequent medical attender or do they have 'thick notes'?

Is there a family history of neurosis?

Notes

- Many people have had neurotic symptoms for years before seeking help. If so, consider personality disorder. Some people view personality disorder as being chronic neurosis.
- Some neuroses have a clear precipitant. If so, the categories of *stress reaction* or *adjustment reaction* apply. Other neuroses are plausibly the result of earlier experience (e.g. a wasp phobia after childhood stings).

• People turn to alcohol and other maladaptive strategies (e.g. avoidance) to cope with anxiety. These need to be identified.

• Assess the disabilities caused by the symptoms — since the presence of dysfunction is one criterion used in the diagnosis of neurosis. For example, are the person's relationships, work or home life affected?

• There is a modest genetic contribution to neurosis, and there may also be relevant learned behaviours from neurotic relatives.

• Finally, remember to assess whether other disorders are present which may explain or coexist with the neurotic symptoms — especially depression.

3.6 Assessment of eating disorders

3.6.1 Using the eating disorder module

This module assesses whether an eating disorder is present and, if so, which one: *anorexia nervosa* or *bulimia nervosa*. When using the module, note that:

• people with eating disorders can be difficult to engage, so take the opportunity to form a good relationship;

• physical complications are frequent and can be serious; and

• the disorders do occur in men.

Triggering the eating disorder module

The eating disorder might be triggered by:

• a patient who says she has problems controlling her eating;

• medically unexplained weight loss;

• a teenage girl with depression and fatigue; or

• a woman who is noted to look thin or is wearing a thick baggy sweater on a hot day.

Related modules

The *depression* and *neurosis* modules will invariably be necessary given the overlap between

these conditions. Use the *substance misuse* module if there is suspicion that drugs are being taken to control weight. Risk assessment is important since deliberate and accidental self-harm can occur.

3.6.2 The eating disorder module

Eating, dieting and bingeing

• Describe a typical day's food intake. Are you dieting?

Ask about weight:

• What is your current weight? How often do you weigh yourself?

• What is your weight history?

Ask about binges:

• Do you ever feel out of control and eat a large amount of food rapidly ('binge')?

• What do you eat in a binge?

• Afterwards, what do you do?

Notes

• A description of a typical day's intake is an informative way of discovering the patient's eating patterns and the quantity and type of food being consumed.

• Dieting in someone who is not overweight should raise suspicion of anorexia nervosa.

• A person's response to being asked about their diet or current weight can itself give clues.

• A past history of obesity and dieting is common in anorexia nervosa.

• Bingeing followed by vomiting is characteristic of bulimia nervosa.

Attitude to weight and shape

• Do you think you are fat? How much would you like to weigh?

• How do you feel about your body? How would you like it to be?

• Do other people say you're too thin? Do you believe them?

• How terrible would it be if you weighed x kilos/stone? (See below.)

Notes

• *Preoccupation with weight and diet* and

distortion of body image are key diagnostic features of anorexia nervosa, so explore fully her views on the subject. The woman may be convinced that she is overweight despite being demonstrably underweight. These beliefs are overvalued ideas rather than delusions or obsessions (p. 12).
- Asking how she would feel if she weighed a normal amount (a body mass index of 18; see below) can be useful.

Physical symptoms of weight loss

Ask about menstrual history. (Check if taking oral contraceptive pill.)
- Are your periods regular? When was your last period?
- When did your periods begin?
- Have you been more tired or weaker than usual recently?

Notes
- Amenorrhoea (or scanty, irregular periods) is a feature of anorexia nervosa. If the disorder began in early teens, menarche may never have occurred.
- Fatigue, lethargy and weakness are consequences of starvation and should alert the doctor to the need for physical examination and investigation.

Additional methods of weight control

Has the patient tried other ways of losing weight?
- What exercise do you do? How often?
- Do you use laxatives, diuretics or slimming pills? Which ones?

Notes
- Misuse of diuretics increases the risk of hypokalaemia.

Physical examination

Weigh the patient and measure them. Calculate the body mass index.
Examine the mouth and hands. Are there callouses? Poor state of teeth?

Check the cardiovascular system.
Note secondary sexual characteristics.
Is there lanugo hair?
Are there signs of past self-mutilation?

Notes
- Patients may wear very baggy clothes, or ensure they have a full bladder, to give a misleading impression of their weight. Weigh them in their underwear.
- The *body mass index (BMI)* is calculated as:

$$\frac{\text{weight}\left(\text{kg}\right)}{\left[\text{height}\left(\text{m}\right)\right]^2}$$

- BMI should be 18–25. In anorexia nervosa, the BMI is below 17.5 — sometimes well below.
- Always examine the *cardiovascular* system. Arrhythmias occur due to hypokalaemia. *Bradycardia* and *peripheral oedema* are common in anorexia.
- There are various signs in the skin, mouth and teeth of people with eating disorder (p. 106).
- Lanugo hair is fine, downy hair on the arms, back and face in anorexia nervosa.
- Self-cutting occurs in a *small* subgroup of people with bulimia nervosa.

Other components of the module

Obtain a history of the development of the eating disorder.
Corroborate history with an informant
Ask about past medical and psychiatric history.
Perform relevant investigations.

Notes
- People with eating disorder often minimize their problems. Always try and confirm the history with regard to dieting, bingeing, etc.
- The differential diagnosis of anorexia nervosa includes inflammatory bowel disease, hypopituitarism and depression.

• Eating disorder is commoner than expected in people with diabetes mellitus.

• Investigations may be needed to rule out other causes of anorexia and weight loss, also to check for *complications* of weight loss: measure electrolytes regularly in anorexia nervosa, especially if history of vomiting, diuretic use or palpitations.

• The core assessment should already have revealed the demographic details associated with increased risk of eating disorder (pp. 106, 109).

3.7 Assessment of substance misuse

3.7.1 Using the substance misuse module

The module aims to establish:

• which substance(s) are used
• the quantity used
• the pattern of consumption
• whether there is dependence or withdrawal
• the associated psychosocial impairment
• the presence of psychiatric and medical complications.

Note that you cannot psychiatrically assess someone who is intoxicated. Though you may be pressured to do so (e.g. by nursing staff in the casualty department), it must be deferred until the person is sober.

Triggering the module

Examples of triggers for this module include:

• Identification of significant alcohol consumption in the core assessment.
• A complaint of insomnia in a stressed and depressed executive.
• Acute psychotic symptoms in a young person.
• Unexplained recurrent episodes of irritability or low mood.

Related modules

The module will be used particularly in associ-ation with the *psychosis, mood* and *cognitive function* modules, given the diagnoses which arise from or coexist with substance misuse. *Risk* assessment is also necessary as substance misusers have high rates of deliberate and accidental self-harm.

3.7.2 The substance misuse module

The questions below refer to alcohol; they should be modified for other substances as necessary.

The quantity and the pattern of consumption

• How much do you drink in the average week? What do you drink?
• Do you sometimes drink much more than that? How often?
• Do you drink every day?

Ask the patient to describe a typical day.
Ask about how long the current pattern has been present.

• When did you start drinking regularly?

Notes

• Self-reports of consumption are underestimates (? by half). The description of a typical day can be more revealing and accurate. It should include the associated behaviours and feelings.
• Check the type of beer drunk — the alcohol content varies considerably.
• Some people misuse alcohol in a steady fashion, others do so in binges.
• Regular drinking which began in early adolescence is common amongst alcohol misusers.
• Ask CAGE questions (p. 10) if not asked already.

Dependence and withdrawal

Ask the patient to rate the importance of drinking compared to other activities.

• Do you have to drink more than you used to in order to get the same effect?
• Have you ever got into trouble because of your drinking?
• Have you ever tried to cut down the amount you drink? What happened?

- Do you feel that you have lost control over your drinking?
- Do you drink more than you intend to?
- Do you ever have a drink in the morning to get you going?

Identify whether the patient continues to drink despite awareness that it is harmful.

Notes
- *Dependence* is a cluster of physiological, behavioural and cognitive features arising from sustained use of alcohol, opioids, amphetamines and some other drugs. It is associated with serious medical and psychiatric complications. Its features include: a *compulsion* to take the substance; *tolerance*—the need for increasing doses of the substance to achieve the same subjective effect; and *withdrawal* symptoms.
- Withdrawal symptoms are a physiological reaction to lack of the substance depended upon, notably alcohol and opioids. Benzodiazapines can produce them as well.
- The symptoms of alcohol withdrawal include tremor, retching, sweating and muscle cramps. If severe, the condition is called *delirium tremens* (p. 140).

Associated psychosocial problems
Ask whether drinking has caused any psychosocial problems.
- Have you got into financial problems because of your drinking?
- Have you had much time off work with hangovers?
- Have you ever lost a job because of your drinking?
- Has it interfered with your relationships?
- Have you ever been in trouble with the police (e.g. drink-driving) because of your drinking?

Notes
- This section is an example of an extended *contextual* history. It is necessary because substance misuse leads to many psychosocial problems.

Psychiatric and medical complications
- Has drinking affected your physical health?
- Have you ever had blackouts while drinking?

Ask about the patient's medical and psychiatric history.

Notes
- Misuse of alcohol and other substances leads to a range of psychiatric and medical disorders, the characteristics of which depend on the substance being misused.
- Psychiatric disorders associated with alcohol misuse include depression, psychosis, delirium and dementia, as well as sexual dysfunction and suicide. Use screening questions from core assessment and then other relevant modules to investigate these areas.

Physical examination
Examine the patient for the stigmata of alcohol dependence.

If the patient has the symptoms or history of a physical illness, examine the appropriate systems.

Notes
- A physical examination is always necessary with alcohol misuse because of its physical effects (p. 140).
- Many medical disorders result from unknown alcohol misuse.
- Opioid use produces its own physical signs (p. 142).
- Needle marks suggest intravenous drug use.

Investigations
Breath alcohol
Full blood count
Liver function tests

Notes

• Medical problems of alcohol misuse suspected from the history or physical examination may need investigation.

• The mean corpuscular volume (MCV) and hepatic γ-glutamyl transpeptidase (γ-GT) are raised in 60–70% of patients with alcohol misuse. If other causes of their elevation are excluded, they are useful as markers of alcohol misuse and for monitoring progress.

• Hepatitis B or HIV testing may be indicated in intravenous users.

Use of other substances

• Have you ever used drugs? What kinds?
• How did you take them?

Notes

• The range of substances which may be encountered are covered in Chapter 14.

• Use similar questions to those used for alcohol to establish the drugs used, the pattern of use and the associated problems.

• Ask about the route of administration because of the additional risks of injection.

3.8 Assessment of the unresponsive patient

3.8.1. Using the unresponsive patient module

By 'unresponsive', we mean a person who does not participate in the assessment. This is uncommon, but causes obvious problems. The module is designed to identify why the person is unable or unwilling to respond.

• We assume that the patient is not unconscious or comatose.

• Because the module is for use when communication is limited, it focuses on the patient's appearance and behaviour, and on a physical examination.

• Where possible, be accompanied. Unresponsive patients can be aggressive, and remember that any examination will be without consent—you may need a witness to confirm what took place.

Triggering the module

By definition, the module will be triggered when a patient does not co-operate with assessment. For example:

• A patient found standing rigidly in the street staring at the sky.

• A patient who does not speak.

• An aggressive patient who does not reply to any questions and demands to leave.

Differential diagnosis

The main diagnostic questions are:

• Is there clouding of consciousness? If so, consider delirium its and various causes (p. 132).

• Is there evidence of psychosis or severe mood disorder? Catatonic schizophrenia and profound depression can both lead to unresponsiveness.

• Does the person seem to be deliberately refusing to co-operate? This may be a sign of malingering or simply due to a belief that they are better off keeping quiet.

• If none of these three apply, consider a dissociative disorder with mutism.

Related modules

Even if the patient is unresponsive it is often possible to use fragments from other relevant modules. Try to assess, however incompletely, *cognitive function, psychosis* and *mood*, and *substance misuse*.

• Complete the assessment when the patient becomes responsive.

3.8.2 The unresponsive patient module

Background information

Is there an informant? Get as many details from them as possible before you start.

• When did the patient become like this?
• Is her condition stable or does it fluctuate?
• Does she feed, dress and toilet herself?

Notes

• If a good informant is available, your problems are largely solved. For example, the patient may be known to have catatonic schizophrenia, to have suffered a recent head injury, or to be wanted by the police.

Level of consciousness

Is the patient responsive to her surroundings?
Ask her to nod or open her eyes.
Does she move?
Do her eyes follow a moving object?
Does she appear to be paying attention to what's going on?

Notes

• Establishing whether there is clouding of consciousness is crucial (p. 13).

• *Stupor* describes a condition in which patient does not speak, move or respond, but appears fully conscious. Amongst psychiatric inpatients, stupor is caused by catatonic schizophenia (30%), depressive disorder (25%), organic disorders such as drug-induced states and akinetic mutism (20%) and dissociative disorder (10%). In other populations (e.g. neurology wards) the proportions — and even the definition of stupor — are different.

• Catatonic stupor in schizophrenia responds, paradoxically, to barbiturates or benzodiazepines. This can be used, with care, as a diagnostic pointer.

Facial expression and communication

Does her expression change?
Does she seem fearful, depressed, preoccupied or hostile?
Does she speak spontaneously or in response to questions?
Can she communicate in other ways, e.g. by writing or hand signals?

Notes

• In elective mutism (p. 161), usually seen in children, the unresponsivity is limited to speaking — other forms of expression and communication are intact.

• Facial expression and behavioural responses give diagnostic clues. For example:

the characteristic appearance of a severely depressed patient;
perplexity and fear in someone with psychosis or delirium;
a severely demented person who seems unaware of your efforts to interview them and sporadically makes irrelevant comments; or
the focused hostility of someone with a personality disorder who does not want to be interviewed.

Motor system

Is posture abnormal? Is it awkward or bizarre?
Is muscle tone normal? Is there resistance when you try and make a movement?
Is there spontaneous movement?
Are there stereotyped movements or mannerisms?

Notes

• These questions are aimed mainly at detecting *catatonia* (p. 20), which usually occurs in catatonic schizophrenia but is also caused by some rare neurological syndromes.

• Increased muscle tone, decreased consciousness and hyperthermia suggests neuroleptic malignant syndrome (Table 7.4, p. 64).

• Surreptitious observation may reveal that the patient behaves differently when unaware she is being observed — indicating that the behaviour is feigned.

Other components of the module

What is the patient's attitude to being examined?
Perform a neurological examination in addition to aspects mentioned above — include cranial nerves, reflexes.
Perform a physical examination — e.g. evidence

of trauma, intoxication, encephalopathy, etc.?

Does the patient have a past psychiatric or medical history?

Following recovery, get patient to describe what he recalls of the period.

Notes

• Examine the neurological system in as much detail as possible. A neurological consultation is worthwhile if no clear psychiatric cause for unresponsiveness is found.

• Check hospital and GP records in case there is a past history.

• After recovery, ask the patient what they recall. For example, someone with catatonic schizophrenia may describe believing that they had to remain motionless in a crucifix position because of a command from God.

CHAPTER 4

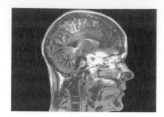

Risk: Harm, Self-Harm and Suicide

4.1 Risk in psychiatry

In psychiatry, *risk* refers to the probability of an adverse event such as self-harm, suicide or harm to others occurring. Increasing public and professional concern about such events makes *risk assessment* and *risk management* an important part of psychiatric practice.

A brief evaluation of risk, especially of suicide, is part of the core assessment, but often a more detailed risk assessment is required, for example in someone with:

• current suicidal intent;
• a history of mood disorder, psychosis or substance misuse; or
• a history of self-harm or violence to others.

This chapter covers the assessment and management of psychiatric risks in general, and the specific issues of self-harm and danger to others.

• Harmful outcomes cannot be eliminated. However, competent risk assessment and management aim to decrease their likelihood.

4.1.1 Risk assessment

Look for features associated with an increased risk of harm.
In the *history*:
• Previous self-harm or harm — the past is the best predictor of the future.
• Recent actions suggestive of impending harm (e.g. buying a hosepipe, making a will).
• Recent major stresses or losses.

• Depressive disorder, psychosis, substance misuse or personality disorder.
In the *mental state*:
• Suicidal or violent thoughts.
• Significant mood disturbance.
• Psychotic symptoms, especially passivity (p. 21).
In the *context*:
• Demographic details (e.g. single men more likely to commit suicide).
• Currently abusing drugs or alcohol.
• Social restlessness — e.g. few relationships, frequent changes of address.
• Easy access to potential weapons or victims.
Try and gather the information from different sources—patient, informants, medical records, social services, police, etc.

Formulation of risk

After completion of risk assessment, document the findings:
• What potential harmful outcome, if any, has been identified?
• What is your estimate of its probability?
• How immediate and long-lasting is the risk?
• What factors may alter the probability?
• What can be done to reduce the risk?

Mr J is referred for a psychiatric opinion because he has threatened to kill his wife and himself. He has convictions for bodily harm and theft. You find no evidence of depressive disorder, psychosis or violent thoughts. However, he admits to drinking heavily at weekends, whereupon he becomes threatening and low in mood. His wife and the police (with his permission) corroborate the history. Your preliminary conclusion is that there is an alcohol-related problem and possibly a personality disorder. His risk of harm or self-harm is low when sober but quite high when intoxicated or stressed. This fluctuating pattern of risk will continue as long as his drinking problem does. Marital strife is the other factor increasing risk.

4.1.2 Risk management
Aims
- Reduce the level of acute risk
- Maintain it at an acceptable level
- Set up a process for reviewing the risk

Management of risk
Divide into immediate and long-term interventions aimed at reducing the risk.
Immediate interventions include:
- Psychiatric admission.
- Use of the Mental Health Act.
- Acute sedation.
- Ensuring there is adequate community support.
- Lowering of tension and provision of reassurance as a result of the assessment itself.
- Making the family and significant others aware of risk.
- Arrest by police.
- Removing access to weapons.
Longer-term interventions include:
- Effectively treating associated psychiatric disorder.
- Implementing a care programme.
- Alleviating psychosocial stresses.
- Enhancing positive coping strategies.
In all cases, ensure that:
- The management plan is documented and communicated to others involved in the case.
- A date is set for reviewing the case and the plan—this may be within hours for an acutely suicidal inpatient, or every 6 months in a stable at-risk patient on the supervision register (p. 81).

You discuss Mr J with your colleagues and draw up a risk management plan. A copy is given to Mr J, his wife and GP. Mr J is given advice to help him cut down his drinking. The couple refer themselves to Relate to try and reduce conflicts between them. It is made clear to Mr J that he will be held responsible should he harm his wife. He agrees to record his alcohol intake and to return in 6 weeks.

4.2 Deliberate self-harm and suicide

4.2.1 Definitions
- *Deliberate self-harm* is the umbrella term for self-injurious behaviours.
- *Attempted suicide* may be used where there was a definite attempt to take one's life, and *parasuicide* when the degree of suicidal intent of the act is not clear.
- *Suicide* is the taking of one's life. Although suicide is clearly defined by death, establishing intent retrospectively is often difficult—some suicides are 'cries for help' which went tragically wrong (e.g. liver failure from untreated paracetamol overdose).

4.2.2 Deliberate self-harm
Deliberate self-harm is important because:
- it is common, accounting for 10% of all acute medical admissions;
- it indicates severe distress and is an opportunity for intervention;
- it is a risk factor for suicide;
- in a minority of cases, it is the presenting feature of serious psychiatric disorder. However, most cases have either a mild depressive disorder, adjustment reaction, personality disorder, or no psychiatric diagnosis.

The motivations to self-harm are various and mixed. Only a few patients have real suicidal intent. Many acts are impulsive, a response to what is perceived as an intolerable situation, or an attempt to influence the behaviour of others. Self-harm is often carried out under the influence of alcohol.

Ms S was seen in casualty having taken 20 paracetamol tablets earlier that night. She had been drinking and had taken them after a row with her *boyfriend. She had not planned to kill herself and now felt foolish about her behaviour. She was unaware that paracetamol could be lethal. She was offered an appointment with a psychiatrist but declined, preferring to see her GP.*

Conversely, deliberate self-harm can reflect a genuine, failed suicide attempt — and a high degree of continuing suicidal intent. Though this is rare, recognition of this group is important, and is one reason for psychiatric assessment of all people presenting after self-harm .

Mr P was found in his fume-filled car in an isolated field and he was resuscitated. He was angry at being saved and still wished to die. He was suffering from psychotic depression and had previously taken a serious overdose. He was admitted under the Mental Health Act and treated with ECT.

4.2.3 Suicide

Suicide accounts for 1% of deaths in the UK, a figure which has fluctuated over the years (Fig. 4.1). Because it affects young people, suicide is the third biggest cause of lost years of life. A Health of the Nation target is to

Fig. 4.1 Number of suicide deaths*, 1911–1990, England and Wales.

reduce rates by 15% by 2000, but recent trends in young men are in the opposite direction (Fig. 4.2).

In most suicides, the attempt is well planned. A common feature is the perception of the future as both intolerable and hopeless. Occasionally this perception may be shared by others (e.g. in terminal cancer), but usually it is strongly biased by depressed mood. The risk factors for suicide are shown in Table 4.1.
• The excess of suicides in the weeks after discharge from psychiatric hospital is clinically important and should be taken into account when planning management.
• In depression, suicide may occur during the initial recovery phase — some people are so depressed that until then they lack the motivation to kill themselves, despite a wish to be dead.
• The increasing suicide rate amongst young men (Fig. 4.2) is unexplained. They rarely have a known psychiatric disorder, though substance misuse may play a role in some.

4.2.4 Assessment of suicide risk

The presence of suicidal risk is routinely determined in the core assessment. If it is found to be present, a full assessment is necessary. This follows the general principles of risk assessment (p. 36), taking into account the

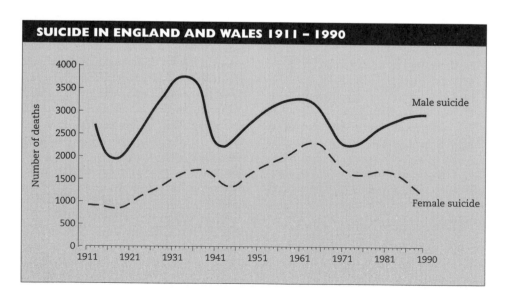

SUICIDE IN ENGLAND AND WALES 1911 – 1990

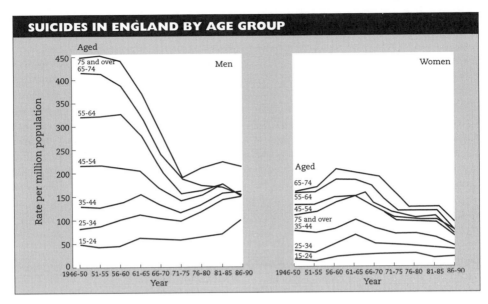

SUICIDES IN ENGLAND BY AGE GROUP

Fig. 4.2 Recorded suicide deaths: rate per million population (by gender and age) 1946–1950 to 1986–1990, England and Wales.

Table 4.1 Risk factors for suicide.

Factor	Comment
Demographic factors	
Male	See Fig. 4.1
Increasing age	See Fig. 4.2
Living alone	
Unemployed	
Recent life crisis	
Occupation	Vets, doctors, nurses, pharmacists and farmers have increased rates
Illness-related factors	
Chronic medical problems	
Psychiatric disorder	Present in 70% of suicide victims, usually depression
Depressive disorder	15% suicide rate in severe depression
Schizophrenia	10% commit suicide
Substance misuse	Especially alcohol and opioid dependence
Personality disorder	Higher suicide rate, especially for borderline type
Previous self-harm	Increases suicide risk 100-fold
Being in psychiatric care	75% of suicides have been in psychiatric treatment
Inpatient	5% of suicides
Recent discharge	See below
Mental state factors	
Depressed mood	See below
Expressed wish to be dead	
Detailed suicide plans	
Hopelessness and helplessness	
Absence of reasons to go on living	E.g. following death of spouse

specific risk factors for suicide (Table 4.1). Particular attention is paid to:

- the person's statements about their immediate intentions;
- their mental state; and
- recent acts of self-harm.

Never omit to assess suicidality because you think: (a) it might precipitate suicide; or (b) someone really planning to kill themselves will deny it. Neither is true — the evidence is that improving recognition may decrease suicide rates.

4.2.5 Assessment following deliberate self-harm

All patients who have self-harmed should be psychiatrically assessed, even if only briefly, to determine their risk of a repeat attempt — within a year 15–20% will do so and 1–2% will commit suicide — and to ascertain if there is an underlying psychiatric disorder.

Certain characteristics of the act are important predictors of suicide:

- The attempt was planned.
- Personal affairs put in order beforehand.
- Took precautions to avoid discovery.
- Did not seek help afterwards.
- Used a method that the patient considered dangerous.
- Left suicide note.

4.2.6 Management of risk of self-harm and suicide

Current risk of suicide

The first priority is to keep the person safe, following the principles of risk management (p. 37).

- Open discussion of the risk and its reduction with the patient is usually possible.
- Keep the person under observation, whether in hospital or by a relative at home.
- Form a positive therapeutic relationship and instil hope.
- Serious suicidal intent is grounds for admission under section 2 of the Mental Health Act, even if the presence of a psychiatric disorder has yet to be established.
- Treat depression effectively.

Patients who repeatedly self-harm

A small number of people, mostly young women, present repeatedly with self-harm from overdoses or wrist cutting. A diagnosis of personality disorder (dramatic cluster; p. 147) is often made, and a history of childhood sexual abuse or other trauma may emerge. Management includes:

- Support which is not triggered by self-harm, to try and reduce any benefits (e.g. increased attention) which the acts produce. A contract may be drawn up whereby a further episode will reduce the level of support.
- Check closely for depressive disorder.

Prevention of suicide

Suicide may be prevented by interventions at the *individual* and at the *social* level. This chapter focuses on the former; the latter requires population-based strategies (Table 4.2).

- A third of people attend their GP in the week preceding suicide — a potential preventative opportunity.

Table 4.2 Prevention of suicide.

Individual interventions
Better detection of suicidal intent
Better detection of depressive disorder
Social interventions
Public education and discussion
Education of doctors and others (e.g. teachers)
Easy, rapid access to psychiatric care or support groups (e.g. Samaritans)
Make it harder to commit suicide
• Limit access to paracetamol — smaller bottles, blister packs
• Make paracetamol safer — include methionine as an antidote
• Make exhaust pipes harder to fix a hose over
• Safety nets around high buildings
Decrease stressors — unemployment, poor housing, etc.

4.3 Risk to others

Psychiatric patients are more likely to be recipients than perpetrators of violence, and most aggressive acts are committed by persons with no psychiatric disorder. Nevertheless, knowing when and how to assess and manage potential harm to others is an important aspect of psychiatric practice.

4.3.1 Assessment of risk to others

The disorders mainly associated with increased risk of violence are substance misuse, schizophrenia and mania, as well as some personality disorders. These disorders act cumulatively—so comorbidity is important to recognize.

• Harmful acts are occasionally due directly to the disorder. For example, passivity experiences in schizophrenia or nihilistic delusions in depression may lead to harm to others without any wilful intent. More commonly, violence results *indirectly* from the same combination of frustrations and personality which determine such acts in anybody. The disorder merely decreases the threshold (and perhaps increases the chances that the aggressor is caught).

• A past history of violence remains the strongest predictor of future violence.

4.3.2 Management of risk to others

After identifying a risk to others, the clinician should do all he or she reasonably can to prevent the harmful outcome. For example, check access to weapons and whether there are specific plans or identified victims.

• The need to warn a potential target can over-ride patient confidentiality, e.g. in morbid jealousy (p. 124).

• If there is known or suspected psychiatric disorder, consider admission, if necessary to a secure unit — discuss with a forensic psychiatrist (p. 79). Conversely, if psychiatric assessment reveals no evidence of psychiatric disorder, this conclusion should be clearly recorded.

4.4 SUMMARY: KEY POINTS

• Risk in psychiatry means risk of harm to self or to others. Assessment of suicide risk should be included in every psychiatric assessment.

• Detection of risk should lead to active management of the risk.

• Deliberate self-harm is very common. All patients who have self-harmed should be screened for suicidal risk and for psychiatric disorder.

• The majority of people committing suicide have depressive disorder or other chronic psychiatric disorder. However, a significant number of suicides occur in young men with no psychiatric history.

• Most psychiatric patients are not violent. Most violence is not committed by psychiatric patients.

• Substance misuse, personality disorder, schizophrenia and mania are all associated with increased risk of harm to others, especially if they coexist.

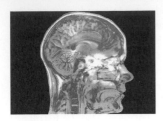

CHAPTER 5

Completing the Assessment, Communicating the Information

5.1 Completing the assessment

The process of psychiatric assessment described in Chapters 2–4 provides diagnostic information and an understanding of the patient's context. These facts are now combined to:
- Make a (differential) diagnosis.
- Identify the factors which have contributed to the disorder.
- Decide your initial management.
- Think about the prognosis.
- Summarize and present the case.

This chapter covers these areas in turn. An overview of the process is given in Fig. 5.1.
- Remember that making a psychiatric diagnosis is not a neutral act—it has drawbacks (e.g. for life insurance, job prospects) as well as benefits (e.g. effective treatment).

5.1.1 The diagnostic process

Assuming the core and module approach has worked, you will have eliminated most possible diagnoses for your patient. Sometimes one overwhelmingly likely diagnosis will remain; usually there is a differential diagnosis which requires further investigation. Either way, draw up a list of the key features in favour of each plausible diagnostic possibility.
- Weighing the diagnostic evidence helps clarify your own thoughts about the case. It's also useful to others who may refer back to

your assessment—for example, if subsequent episodes lead to a review of the diagnosis.
- Throughout the chapter, we will use a single vignette to show how different aspects of a case are highlighted depending on the stage in the diagnostic process and the clinical situation.

Mr K, aged 50, has been referred after a suicide attempt. You have elicited many depressive symptoms, some anxiety symptoms and alcohol intake of ~40 units/week. There are no features suggestive of psychosis or personality disorder. Your provisional diagnosis is depressive disorder, plus alcohol misuse.

It is now time to add in the contextual information collected during the core and modules, particularly those factors which appear to help explain the origins and evolution of the disorder.

5.2 The context and cause of the case

When considering causative factors in psychiatry, the two key variables are:
- the *type* of factor. These are best divided into biological, psychological and social.
- the *time* at which the factor operates. A useful mnemonic is predisposing, precipitating and perpetuating ('the three Ps').

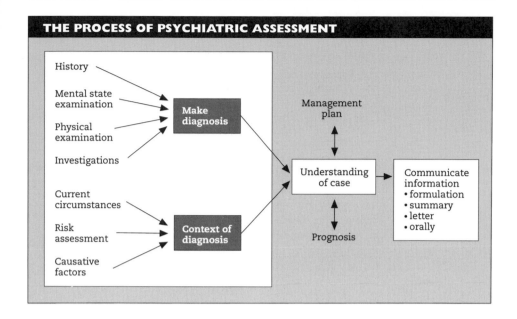

THE PROCESS OF PSYCHIATRIC ASSESSMENT

Fig. 5.1 The process of psychiatric assessment.

5.2.1 Biological, psychological and social factors

The development of psychiatric disorders is influenced by biological (genetic and environmental), psychological and social factors (Chapter 6). Sometimes one predominates, sometimes another.

We return to Mr K. He became unemployed 6 months ago. He is gay and his partner left him 3 months ago, after which he had several casual homosexual encounters. He has no close friends or relatives. Mr K had a stroke last year which left him with a mild hemiparesis. He has had two past depressive episodes. His father committed suicide when Mr K was 5.

In this case, the putative causative factors for his probable depressive disorder are:

Biological
• Genetic predisposition (? his father had a depressive disorder).
• His stroke (associated with depressive disorder).
• Alcohol misuse (associated with depressive disorder).
• ?? HIV.

Psychological
• Stress of being gay (? a secret, ? a source of conflict).
• Recent breakdown of a serious relationship.
• ? Guilt about recent sexual liaisons.

Social
• Social isolation (? his stroke has stopped him driving).
• ? His unemployment is causing him worry or financial stress.

Having hypothesized causal factors, try and substantiate them. For example, in this case:
• examine for neurological deficits;
• find out more about his alcohol misuse;
• discover his views on his sexuality;
• suggest an HIV test, with counselling;
• investigate why he was made redundant and how he feels about it;

• get hold of his case notes and review his earlier depressive episodes;
• get hold of his father's psychiatric case notes.

You find that Mr K has only minimal physical impairment. He has misused alcohol intermittently for many years; the recent increase in consumption seems to have been a response to his low mood. His sexuality conflicts with his religious beliefs. He feels he was made redundant unfairly because he had taken sick leave, and has been left with serious financial problems. He is HIV negative. His notes reveal a similar picture during previous episodes, with a good response to ECT and antidepressants. His father's case notes are lost (this is a realistic vignette!). You conclude that he has a recurrent depressive disorder.

The biopsychosocial model
Biological, psychological and social factors always contribute something to each disorder. Hence the *biopsychosocial model* of psychiatry, in which due attention is paid to all three and which encourages an equally eclectic approach to therapy.
• The model should seem obvious and essential. However, psychiatry has at times been guilty of focusing too closely on one or other of its components. This has led to 'mindless' psychiatrists (who see only the molecules) and 'brainless' psychiatrists (who see only the minds and the social issues). We hope we are neither, but we could be both.

5.2.2 Predisposing, precipitating and perpetuating factors
In terms of timing, causal factors can be:
• *Predisposing*—those which exert a long-term or distant causal effect, such as genetic make-up and early childhood experiences.
• *Precipitating*—factors which explain why the disorder has occurred now. They include life events as well as other factors such as discontinuing medication.
• *Perpetuating* — factors affecting the course of a disorder. Marital problems and non-adherence to treatment are two common

ones. The nature of the disorder itself is also relevant; for example, Alzheimer's disease requires no perpetuating factors.

In these terms, the causative factors for Mr K's depression would be:

Predisposing	Genetic predisposition
	Psychological effects of father's suicide
	Guilt about his sexuality
	Alcohol misuse
	Stroke
	Past history of depression
Precipitating	Ending of long-term relationship
	Increased alcohol intake
	Being made redundant
Perpetuating	Social isolation
	Stresses continue
	Alcohol intake

• The same factor (in this case alcohol) can be involved in all three aspects of aetiology.

5.2.3 Summarizing the causative factors
Combining the biopsychosocial and 'three Ps' approaches leads to a 3 × 3 box. The box may be used literally (and included in the case notes) or metaphorically (as another *aide-mémoire*). A 3 × 3 box for Mr K is shown in Fig. 5.2.

Life charts
An alternative way to clarify the role of different causal factors is a *life chart*. This is most useful when the history is long and complex, to show whether episodes can be related to specific factors, and whether there is any pattern of treatment response.
• A life chart is time consuming but usually worthwhile — and always impressive.

5.2.4 The future context
Once you have (a) made a diagnosis and (b) investigated the causative factors, it's time to

CAUSATION IN PSYCHIATRY: THE EXAMPLE OF Mr K.

	Predisposing	Precipitating	Perpetuating
Biological	Genetic predisposition Alcohol misuse Past history of depression	Stroke Increased alcohol intake	Effects of stroke Effects of alcohol
Psychological	Effect of father's suicide Guilt/stress about his sexuality	Relationship breakdown Guilt about recent sexual liaisons	Unresolved relationship issues Continuing guilt
Social	Childhood deprivation	Social isolation Unemployment	Continuing isolation Financial worries

Fig. 5.2 A 3 × 3 box for patient Mr K.

consider the *management* and *prognosis* — the 'future context' — since these follow directly from your current understanding of the case, and both will be mentioned in the summary, letter or phone call which arises from the assessment.

Fig. 5.3 A life chart for Mr K, 2 years later. By this time his depressive disorder has resolved, for one of several plausible reasons.

Management

Management in psychiatry involves making a number of decisions, several of which need to be made after the initial assessment. For example:

• *Does the person need treatment?* Some assessments produce no evidence of psychiatric disorder and no indication for treatment — just reassurance and a clear statement of your conclusions.

• *How urgent is the problem?* Acute psychosis and severe mood disorders generally need immediate treatment. Serious risk of self-harm

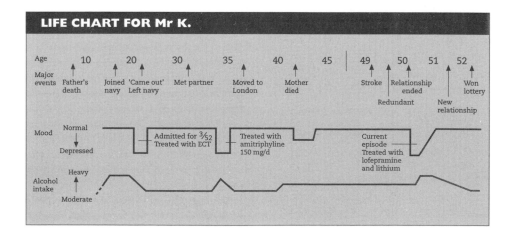

LIFE CHART FOR Mr K.

or harm to others is a major determinant of urgency. Is the patient sufficiently ill or at risk to need compulsory treatment?

• *Where should treatment take place, and by whom?* Most psychiatric disorders are treated by GPs; some will be referred to psychiatrists; a few need admission (Fig. 18.1, p. 171).

• *What management is indicated?* Treatment decisions depend, of course, on the diagnosis. However, they are also affected by the context — another reason why contextual information was collected in the assessment. For example, is he motivated enough for a psychological treatment? Should I avoid sedative antidepressants?

Prognosis

Once you have a diagnosis and a reasonable understanding of the person's history and circumstances, a provisional judgement about prognosis should be possible.

• Together with the diagnosis, prognosis is the information which the patient, their relatives and the referrer are most interested in.

Short-term prognosis depends mainly on the natural history of the disorder and, particularly, the treatment response. It is usually possible to give a rough estimate of the likelihood of improvement and its timing. For example, someone with a depressive episode who takes an antidepressant is likely (60% chance) to be significantly better in 2 months (p. 58).

Long-term prognosis is much more difficult to predict, and opinion on this issue may be deferred. There are several non-specific factors which apply to most disorders, and which identify people at higher risk of a poor outcome:

• Insidious onset.
• Longer duration of disorder prior to treatment.
• Coexistent personality disorder.
• Coexistent substance misuse.
• Lack of close relationships.
• History of poor adherence to treatment.

5.3 Summarizing and communicating cases

In the assessment process, you have generated and tested diagnostic hypotheses, collected contextual information and, in parallel, have considered the management and prognosis. Your understanding of the case must now be shared with others, including the GP and other agencies currently involved, and those who may use the information in the future. Here we illustrate four ways of presenting psychiatric information — a case formulation, a case summary, a problem list and a letter to a GP.

When planning a psychiatric communication, ask yourself:

• *What does the recipient want to know?* This can vary from a detailed discharge summary for the psychiatric case notes to a brief letter informing a GP that the dose of a drug has been changed. Avoid unnecessary information — it hinders the reader from attending to the important bits. On the other hand, always include important negatives (e.g. 'He is not suicidal.' 'Her urine drug screen was negative.'). Similar rules apply to oral presentations.

• *What does the recipient know already?* If you're summarizing a person's tenth admission, information about the previous nine is likely to be available to and known by everyone involved, and need not be repeated. Conversely, a psychiatric court report should be written assuming the recipient knows nothing about the person, and nothing about psychiatry.

5.3.1 The psychiatric formulation

The formulation is a concise, informative way of summarizing a psychiatric assessment. It is also educational, since it involves weighing up the evidence and showing how you came to your conclusions. The formulation consists of:

• *Opening statement* — patient's name, age, occupation, presenting complaint and main findings.

• *Differential diagnosis.* Put the most likely first. Include the factors for and against each diagnosis. Remember that more than one diagnosis may be needed (comorbidity; p. 4).

• *Context and cause*—summarize the causative factors and relevant context. This can be done in different ways (p. 45) — choose one which suits you and the case.

• *Management plan.* Include investigations and immediate interventions.

• *Prognosis.*

Example of formulation
(As might be produced for a ward round following admission.)

Opening statement
Mr K is a 50-year-old ex-electrician. He presented following an overdose and was admitted voluntarily because of suicidal intent and many depressive symptoms. Relevant factors included recent redundancy, break up of his long-term homosexual relationship, and alcohol misuse.

Differential diagnosis
1 *Depressive disorder. In favour: subjectively and objectively low mood, suicidal ideation, recent self-harm, poor sleep, loss of appetite, feelings of guilt and worthlessness; two prior depressive episodes. Against:? his depressive symptoms are secondary to diagnoses 2–4.*
2 *Anxiety disorder. In favour: worrying about his health, feeling tense, socially phobic, and lies awake worrying. Against: the depressive symptoms began first, and are clearly more prominent.*
3 *Alcohol misuse. In favour: drinking 40+ units/week; long history of harmful intake; describes withdrawal symptoms when in the navy (30 years ago). Against: intake over past few years has averaged 25 units/week; recent increase postdated onset of symptoms; normal LFTs and MCV.*
4 *Organic mood disorder. In favour: stroke last year. Against: this seems insufficient to explain his symptoms; no focal neurological signs; preceding history of depressive disorder.*

Context and cause
Predisposing factors. Father had depression and committed suicide when Mr K aged 5. Alcohol misuse. Guilt about his sexuality. Stroke last year. Two other depressive episodes (ages 22, 34).
Precipitating factors. His partner left him 3 months ago after 20 years. Increased alcohol intake. Made redundant 6 months ago.
Perpetuating factors. Social isolation — no close friends or family. Feeling guilty about recent casual homosexual affairs — and worried about risk of HIV. Continuing high alcohol intake. Financial worries.

Management plan
1 *Further investigations: repeat LFTs; HIV test; get old notes; phone GP for background.*
2 *Monitor mental state daily. Continue nursing observations whilst actively suicidal.*
3 *Observe for signs of alcohol withdrawal.*
4 *Start antidepressant [specify drug and dose]. Benzodiazepine as required for sedation.*
5 *As mental state settles, assess further the current stressors—employment, finance, sexuality.*
6 *Longer term will need continuing support — begin care programme approach assessment [p. 80].*

Prognosis
His history predicts a good response to antidepressants. However, if stresses continue, recovery will be compromised and he will be vulnerable to relapse.

5.3.2 Case summaries
A psychiatric case summary is equivalent in most respects to a medical one. It is useful:
• at the end of a psychiatric admission;
• at discharge from psychiatric care; and
• when the patient is being transferred to other psychiatric services.

Suggested headings are shown in Table 5.1 — they overlap with those of the core assessment (p. 9).
• As an exercise, summarize Mr K's case in this format.

5.3.3 Problem lists
Once the background to a case is familiar, the emphasis usually switches to current problems and their solution. *Problem lists*

Table 5.1 Headings for a psychiatric case summary.

Demographic details
   Name, age, sex, occupation, presenting
     complaint
   Dates of: referral, assessment, admission,
     discharge,
   Mental Health Act status
History of presenting complaint
   Onset, progression, treatments to date
Past psychiatric history
   Diagnoses, admissions, treatments
Personal history
   Childhood, academic and job record,
     relationships, children
   Premorbid personality
Use of alcohol and drugs
Mental state examination
   Key symptoms present and absent
Risk assessment
Physical examination
Investigations
Differential diagnosis
Management and progress to date
   Rationale and outcome of interventions
   Current symptoms and problems
Future management plans
Prognosis

ensure that the key issues are identified and dealt with.

Mr K's problem list (at the time of the formulation on p. 47) might read thus:

5.3.4 Writing to GPs

Letters from psychiatrists to GPs should be as concise as possible. Remember that the GP will often know at least as much as you about the person's history and circumstances. Take into account the purpose of the referral: was it for an opinion or continuing care? Has the GP asked a specific question or requested a particular intervention? Generally the GP is most interested in:

• Your formulation of the case, including a clear diagnosis.

• A specific management plan, including the date of review.

• What the patient/relative has been told.

• What the patient and GP should do if matters unexpectedly deteriorate.

As a final visit to Mr K's case, here is a letter recording his discharge back to the GP's care.

Dear Dr,

re: Mr J.K., dob 1.1.47, 24 Easy Street, Anytown
Diagnosis: severe depressive disorder

Mr K has made a good recovery from his illness which was detailed in the discharge summary sent to you in February. He has no residual symptoms but is understandably anxious about relapse.

Table 5.2 Problem list for patient Mr K.

Problem	Action	Agent	Review
Depressive disorder	Start amitriptyline 50 mg	Psychiatrist	One week — plan to increase dose
Suicide risk	Close observation	Nursing staff	Daily
Social isolation	Investigate supports	Social worker	One week
Guilt about homosexuality	Get contact number of local gay Christian group	Social worker	One week
HIV status	1 Counselling for HIV test 2 Standard precautions	Psychiatrist	Two weeks
Alcohol misuse	Counselling (when mental state improved)	Specialist nurse	Unspecified

Thank you for prescribing his antidepressants (amitriptyline 150 mg nocte; lithium carbonate 800 mg nocte), which he has taken as prescribed. His lithium level will need to be checked in 6 weeks and maintained at 0.5–0.8 mmol/l — it was stable at 0.72 mmol/l last week. He should continue the medication for another 6 months, at which time it should be gradually tailed off.

Mr K is fully aware of the diagnosis and our formulation of its causes (especially the relationship break-up, guilt about his sexuality, and the increased alcohol intake). We have addressed these issues and they appear largely resolved. His drinking is now minimal and his LFTs have remained normal. Also on the positive side, he is in a new and seemingly stable relationship, and his financial worries have evaporated having won a large sum on the national lottery.

We have not arranged to see him again. Please feel free to get in touch if you wish to discuss his case further.

5.4 SUMMARY: KEY POINTS

- Completing the psychiatric assessment involves:
  - using the information you have collected to make a diagnosis and to plan management; and
  - evaluating the factors which have caused the disorder.
- When thinking about causation, divide the factors according to their timing and type into:
  - predisposing, precipitating and perpetuating; and biological, psychological and social.
- A formulation is a useful way of summarizing a psychiatric case. It comprises: an introductory statement; the evidence for and against each differential diagnosis; the causative factors; the management plan; and the prognosis.
- Tailor the content and format of any communication to the needs of the recipient. Be concise and structured, and emphasize the points relevant to diagnostic and management decisions.

CHAPTER 6

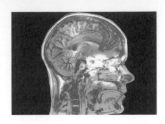

Aetiology

6.1 Aetiological factors in psychiatry

Chapter 5 included an introduction to causation because understanding how and why a person's disorder has occurred is an integral part of the psychiatric assessment. In this chapter we examine general issues of psychiatric aetiology.
• Aetiological conclusions should be just as evidence-based as therapeutic and diagnostic ones.

6.1.1 Causation in psychiatry

Apart from a few familial dementias due to single gene mutations, psychiatric disorders are caused by multiple and diverse influences— some known, some unknown. No one factor is necessary or sufficient, and one causal factor can contribute to several different disorders. It is therefore best to think in terms of multiple and overlapping risk factors. For example, we might attribute a teenager's eating disorder to:
• inheritance of a genetic predisposition;
• childhood obesity;
• wanting to be a ballerina;
• peer, parental or societal pressure to be thin;
• disturbed 5-HT neurotransmission; or
• a hypothalamic tumour.
  Approaches to the study of aetiology in psychiatry have to be equally wide ranging, as summarized in Table 6.1 and reviewed in turn.

6.2 Epidemiology

Epidemiology is a tool which can be applied to social, psychological or biological studies. It has contributed in two main ways to psychiatry:
• Population surveys have provided good information about the *prevalence* and *incidence* of the major psychiatric disorders, their sex and age distribution, and so on.
• Cohort and case control studies have identified *risk factors* for psychiatric disorders. For example, it has been found that head injury doubles the risk of dementia. Sometimes, as in this example, the causality of an epidemiological finding is clear, but often it is not (e.g. the association of unemployment with depression), and further studies must be carried out to see which way the causal arrows point.

6.3 Social models

Social factors are important in both the cause and the shaping of psychiatric disorder. They can operate at different levels:
• *The immediate physical environment.* One's surroundings act as non-specific risk factors for illness. For example, psychiatric (and medical) disorders are twice as common in those living in deprived conditions. Many mechanisms are involved, including social conflict, substance misuse, noise and over-

Table 6.1 Approaches to studying the aetiology of psychiatric disorders.

Field	Approaches
Epidemiology	Prevalence and incidence studies Risk factor studies
Sociology	Life events Family influences Cultural factors Illness behaviour
Psychology	Behavioural theories Cognitive theories Psychodynamic theories Personality theories Neuropsychology
Biology	Genetics Biochemistry and pharmacology Brain structure Animal models

crowding; there may also be factors which contribute independently to poverty and psychiatric disorder. In addition, having a psychiatric disorder may make it harder for the person to improve their circumstances and make continuing poverty more likely.
• *The social and family group.* Parents, siblings and others close to us are important influences on our development and functioning, for better and worse. For example, childhood emotional deprivation predisposes to depression, whereas being in a close relationship protects against the effect of stressors. Some familial influence is genetic, some environmental.
• *The wider environment.* Environment in a broader sense is also relevant. For example, society's attitudes to beauty and body shape contribute to the prevalence of eating disorders, whilst political decisions affect the types and quantities of substances misused. Sociologists have also investigated *transcultural* differences in the occurrence of psychiatric disorders — some appear to be universal (e.g.

schizophrenia), others specific for particular populations (p. 97).

6.3.1 Life events

Life events are specific stressors. They include marriage, bereavement, unemployment and moving house. Life events, especially negative ones, lead to an increased risk of psychiatric disorder, notably depression, in the succeeding months.
• Where a life event is the predominant and understandable trigger for a psychiatric disorder, the diagnostic category of *stress reaction* or *adjustment reaction* is used (p. 100).

6.3.2 The social origins of depression

A classic example of the role of social factors in psychiatry concerns depressive disorder. Researchers wondered why depression was particularly common in women of low socioeconomic status, and why some women did not get depressed despite similar circumstances. They identified several factors:
• Women who as children had suffered emotional deprivation or the death of a parent were at greater risk of depression. Other *vulnerability (predisposing) factors* included not having a supportive partner or close friend, and being stuck at home with several young children.
• In the women to whom one or more of the vulnerability factors applied, depressive disorder was *precipitated* by a single major life event or by an accumulation of minor stressors.
• Continuing stress and lack of support acted as *perpetuating* factors.
A similar combination of social factors is now known to be associated with depression in other environments and groups.

On occasion, the causal role of social factors has been overemphasized. For example, people with schizophrenia are more likely to be of low social class and to live in inner cities, factors which were interpreted as being specific contributors to schizophrenia. This was wrong for two reasons:

• Social deprivation is associated with psychiatric and medical morbidity in general.
• The social class and geographical distribution of the parents of people with schizophrenia are unremarkable; the findings reflect a drift of people with schizophrenia down the social scale and into deprived areas.

6.3.3 Family theories

Family theories view psychiatric disorder in one member as reflecting an abnormality in the family itself. They are applied particularly to childhood psychiatric disorders, where the theories have inspired a treatment approach— *family therapy* (p. 71). However, it has been hard to confirm the aetiological role of the family, for two main reasons:

• Recent research shows that resemblances between family members are more influenced by genes than by shared environment. An example where family factors (in a sociological sense) were wrongly invoked is autism, which was attributed to parents being aloof or obsessional but in fact is a highly genetic disorder (p. 159).
• How do you show that family abnormalities are causal? In the 1950s, schizophrenia was explained in terms of parenting styles (the 'schizophrenogenic mother') and patterns of family communication ('double bind'; 'schism and skew'). Such abnormalities, if they occur, seem more likely to be the result of having a schizophrenic relative in the house or of shared genes (i.e. the relatives have a partially expressed phenotype of schizophrenia).

6.3.4 The sick role and illness behaviour

The *sick role* describes four processes that occur when someone is ill:

1 exemption from normal obligations (such as earning a living);
2 a right to receive care;
3 an obligation to co-operate with care; and
4 a desire to recover.

Illness behaviour refers to the behaviour of the person in the sick role.

Both the sick role and illness behaviour are sociological concepts which describe normal processes. They can also be maladaptive, so becoming relevant to the understanding of the presentation and persistence of psychiatric disorders.

• People differ markedly in their response to symptoms — they vary in their illness behaviour and readiness to adopt the sick role. Some are stoical and are reluctant to see a doctor, others dramatize symptoms and have a low threshold for medical consultation. These individual differences are compounded by society's views about psychiatric disorder — including stigma and ignorance about their nature and treatability. As a result, psychiatric patients have more difficulty than medical patients negotiating a sick role for themselves.
• Patients with medical complaints who appear to adopt the sick role unnecessarily or excessively (i.e. have *abnormal illness behaviour*) may have depression or a somatoform disorder (p. 101 and p. 172).
• The benefits of the sick role (sometimes called *secondary gain*) play an especially important role in dissociative disorders (p. 101).

6.3.5 Antipsychiatry

Some sociologists, and even a few psychiatrists, have argued that psychiatric disorders are simply social constructs to deal with deviant behaviour, reinforced by psychiatrists to legitimize their existence. This thesis — *antipsychiatry* — was influential in the 1960s. Whilst antipsychiatry was important in drawing attention to the limitations of psychiatric knowledge and the dangers of stigmatization and institutionalization, there is little evidence to support it, and it is not helpful to patients.

6.4 Psychological models

There are various psychological models of psychiatric disorder, differing in their theoretical background and experimental support, but sharing two features:

• They are extensions of theories of normal psychological processes.

• There is a psychological treatment based upon the theory.

6.4.1 Behavioural theories

Many of our actions are explicable in terms of learned behaviours or *conditioning*. There are two types of conditioning, *classical* and *operant*. These underlie contemporary *behavioural theories* of normal and abnormal behaviours.

• Behavioural theories have given rise to *behavioural therapy*, an effective intervention for several psychiatric disorders (p. 67).

Classical conditioning

In classical conditioning, we unconsciously associate two stimuli which regularly occur together. In Pavlov's famous experiments, dogs were given food when a bell was rung. After a while the dogs began to salivate when the bell rang, even if no food was there. This conditioning gradually wears off (*extinction*).

We are classically conditioned in many ways: we learn to relax when the theme tune to *Neighbours* is heard, and men become aroused at the sight of lingerie (if they have come to associate it with impending sexual gratification). Conditioning is important in the development of some psychiatric disorders. For example, agoraphobia developing in a woman who has been twice assaulted in the street; she associates leaving the house with the fear of attack, which she avoids by staying at home.

Operant conditioning

Operant conditioning results from the fact that a behaviour occurs more frequently if it is rewarded (*positive reinforcement*), and decreases if it is not (*negative reinforcement*) or if it has unpleasant consequences (*punishment*). Rats learn to press a lever if it gives them food, but not to press it if it doesn't or if they receive a painful shock. Children will shout and scream if they learn that this behaviour gets them an ice-cream; on the other hand, they learn to be polite if that is effective in obtaining an ice-cream. Adults are equally conditionable, though we might not like to think so.

• *Learned helplessness* is an example of operant conditioning. Young animals subjected to inescapable stresses (electric shocks) grow up to become animals who give up easily on tasks, whereas those given shocks from which they can escape become adults who carry on and solve the same tasks. In other words, the latter group learns that solving problems is possible, the former group learns that it isn't. A similar mechanism is proposed to explain why childhood adversity predisposes to depression in adulthood.

6.4.2 Cognitive theories

The core assumption of cognitive theories is that cognitions (thoughts and ways of processing information) influence our mood, behaviour and physiology, and that inaccurate or distorted cognitions can lead to inappropriate or abnormal mood and behaviour.

• Cognitive theories of depressive disorder and panic disorder are especially well developed.

A woman gets a twinge of chest pain whilst reaching for a tin of beans in the supermarket. She has the thought that it might be a heart attack and remembers her father died of one. She becomes more anxious and develops the physiological changes associated with anxiety (p. 98). She interprets these sensations as confirming that she is having a heart attack, the anxiety increases, and she has a panic attack. The next time she is in the supermarket she recalls the episode, becomes hypervigilant for bodily sensations, and a second panic attack occurs more readily than before. As the cycle continues, her cognitions and the associated symptoms are repeated until she has established panic disorder.

The cognitive model explaining how panic disorder develops is summarized in Fig. 6.1.

• In the equivalent cognitive model of depression, the central abnormality is dysfunctional assumptions and negative thoughts which lead

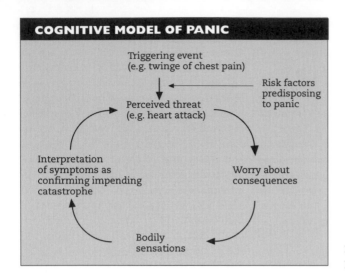

COGNITIVE MODEL OF PANIC

Fig. 6.1 Cognitive model of a panic attack.

to a vicious cycle of lowered mood and more negative thoughts.

• Cognitive distortions can arise for different reasons. For example, the lady above may be at risk of panic because of a genetic predisposition or a history of asthma, or because she had drunk too much strong coffee that morning.

• Cognitive theories are well validated and are clinically important because they have led to an effective form of psychotherapy — *cognitive therapy* (p. 68).

6.4.3 Psychodynamic theories
Psychoanalysis
Psychoanalysis is a complex theory of psychological processes and the origins of psychiatric disorders, especially neurosis. Psychoanalysis has changed a lot since the time of Freud and the generic term *psychodynamic* is usually used to describe theories which combine Freudian elements with later ideas.

Psychodynamic theory includes the following features:

• Psychoanalysis is both a theory and a therapy.

• Feelings and memories of which we are unaware, especially those arising early in life, shape our current thoughts and feelings.

• The mind is partitioned; some is conscious but much is unconscious. In Freud's final model, the components of the mind were the ego, superego and id: the ego is the part of us in contact with reality; the superego is our conscience; and the id is our instinctive drives and desires. The id's energy is called *libido*, which is primarily sexual in nature.

• Neuroses result from a failure to progress through normal stages of mental development.

• We use unconscious *defence mechanisms* to reduce tensions which exist between our conflicting desires (Table 6.2). These mechanisms may be healthy or dysfunctional.

The status of psychodynamic theories
Psychodynamic theories have been influential but have declined in importance for several reasons:

• They are not scientific theories—it is hard to test or refute them.

• When elements of the theories have been tested they have not been supported by evidence.

• Psychodynamic psychotherapies are of unproven, perhaps unprovable, efficacy.

Nevertheless, psychodynamic insights are still clinically useful in three areas:

Table 6.2 Some Freudian defence mechanisms.

Defence mechanism	Definition
Repression	Suppressing desires and memories from consciousness
Denial	Behaving as though genuinely unaware of external reality
Projection	Attributing your own feelings to someone else
Displacement	Shifting emotions from the appropriate object or person to a more acceptable (less unpleasant) target. For example, kicking the dog rather than your father
Reaction formation	Behaving in a way opposite to your (unacceptable) instincts
Regression	Regressing to an earlier pattern of behaviour. For example, becoming more dependent on others to cope with an insoluble problem
Sublimation	Finding a socially acceptable alternative outlet for emotions
Intellectualization	Thinking about your desires rather than feeling them

• Emphasizing that early experiences and unconscious processes affect our feelings and actions.
• Psychological defence mechanisms (Table 6.2).
• *Transference* and *countertransference* (p. 69) are relevant to the doctor–patient relationship.

6.4.4 The role of personality
Personality describes our persistent pattern of thoughts, attitudes and behaviours. As such, it is inextricably linked to psychiatric disorder, but the very fact that the two are so intertwined makes it hard to identify the specific aetiological relationships between them. It is clear, though, that:
• Different personality types predispose to different psychiatric disorders.
• Personality affects the clinical picture of psychiatric disorder (i.e. acts as a *pathoplastic* factor).
• Personality affects the prognosis of psychiatric disorders.
These issues are discussed in Chapter 15.

6.5 Biological models

6.5.1 Genetics
A genetic contribution to a psychiatric disor-

der may be suspected for one of three reasons:
• If the disorder clusters in families. Familial aggregation can be shown to reflect shared genes not shared environment if the incidence of the disorder remains increased in adopted-away children, and if monozygotic twins have higher concordance rates than dizygotic twins.
• If there is a known chromosomal (*cytogenetic*) aberration — e.g. Down's syndrome (p. 166).
• If there is a known pathological or biochemical abnormality, the underlying gene is a *candidate gene* for the disorder. For example, in Alzheimer's disease, the β-amyloid protein in senile plaques led to the discovery of amyloid gene mutations (p. 127). The lack of definitive lesions in most psychiatric disorders means there are few convincing candidate genes.

Although a genetic contribution has been established for many psychiatric disorders, it is proving difficult to complete the next step (Fig. 6.2) — location of the chromosomal loci and causative genes — despite using the molecular techniques being applied successfully elsewhere in medicine. There are several possible reasons for this slow progress:
• There are probably many genes, each conferring a small amount of the risk for a psychiatric disorder. If so, the genes will be hard to find,

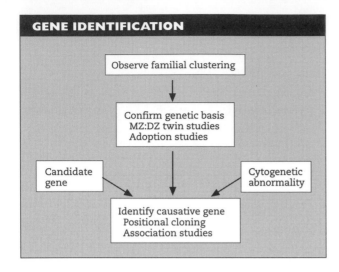

Fig. 6.2 Finding genes for psychiatric disorders.

and population genetic association studies (looking for genetic variants associated with a differential risk) are most likely to reveal them.
• Whilst there may be a major gene, a second gene or an environmental factor may also be needed — a *two-hit* model.
• The disorder may be caused by different genes in different people (*genetic heterogeneity*).
• The causative genes may not map onto the currently defined clinical syndromes. That is, the wrong patients, genetically speaking, are being grouped together.

6.5.2 Biochemistry and pharmacology
Biochemical theories propose that psychiatric disorders are caused by a disturbance in the level or activity of an enzyme, neurotransmitter or receptor.
• Some theories are based on the mechanisms by which psychotropic drugs work. For example, antipsychotics treat schizophrenia and were found to block dopamine receptors; this observation led to the dopamine hypothesis of schizophrenia (p. 121). This line of reasoning is flawed: diuretics treat heart failure, but heart failure is not usually due to renal disease.

Measurements in the brain
Biochemical studies of the brain were crucial in the development of our understanding of Alzheimer's disease; in particular, the discovery of cholinergic deficits (p. 127) and the β-amyloid protein. Similar approaches have revealed abnormalities in schizophrenia and mood disorders, but no clear picture has emerged.
• Studies of post-mortem brains have many limitations, such as the effects of dying and death, and a bias towards old, medicated, chronically ill cases. This makes it difficult to establish whether alterations occurred early or late in the disease, and to exclude the effects of ageing or treatment.

Functional imaging overcomes these problems. It allows first-episode and unmedicated subjects to be studied. Various imaging modalities are being applied:
• Positron emission tomography (PET) and single photon emission tomography (SPET) use radioactive ligands to measure brain receptors. They have shown, for example, that people with schizophrenia do not have elevated dopamine D_2 receptors (as one version of the dopamine hypothesis had proposed).
• PET, SPET and functional magnetic resonance imaging (fMRI) can be used to measure

regional brain metabolism and cerebral activity. Such information points to brain regions which may be involved in the pathophysiology of a disorder.

Peripheral markers
The brain is relatively inaccessible, so many biochemical measurements have been made in cerebrospinal fluid (CSF), blood or urine. A robust finding is that people who are impulsive and aggressive have low CSF levels of the metabolite of 5-HT, suggesting impaired functioning of the central 5-HT system.

• In a *neuroendocrine challenge test*, a substance known to produce a change in the plasma level of a hormone is administered. The size of the change is used as a marker of the sensitivity of the system which mediates the response in the brain.

• In the dexamethasone suppression test (DST), plasma cortisol is measured after a dose of dexamethasone, to assess hypothalamic–pituitary–adrenal (HPA) axis function. Many people with severe depression fail to suppress cortisol — leading to a 'steroid hypothesis' of depression.

6.5.3 Brain structure
Neuropathology
Most psychiatric disorders do not have a known neuropathological basis. Nevertheless, recent studies using sensitive and molecular techniques suggest that there may be histolog-ical changes in schizophrenia (p. 122) and autism, and perhaps in other psychiatric disorders also.

Structural brain imaging
Computed tomography (CT) and MRI allow brain structure to be investigated *in vivo*. For example, they show that patients first presenting with schizophrenia already have enlarged lateral ventricles, and that mood disorder in the elderly is associated with abnormalities in the white matter.

6.5.4 Animal models
No one would suggest that a rat can get schizophrenia — and how would we know if it did? However, animal studies have contributed to psychiatric research in various ways — Pavlov and learned helplessness have already been mentioned.

• Studies are used to assess the effects of an experimental intervention (e.g. maternal separation, neonatal hippocampal damage) upon relevant behaviours (e.g. cognitive performance, social interactions) and biology (e.g. receptor sensitivity).

• *Transgenic* animals allow the role of specific genes in brain function and dysfunction to be investigated. For example, mice containing a mutated human amyloid precursor protein gene develop cognitive impairment and histological features of Alzheimer's disease.

6.6 SUMMARY: KEY POINTS

• The cause of most psychiatric disorders is multifactorial. It involves biological, psychological and social factors.

• There is a definite but moderate genetic predisposition to most disorders. The number and nature of the genes involved remain unknown.

• Other biological factors include head injury, drugs and viral infections.

• Important psychological factors are cognitive style and conditioning.

• Social influences include childhood deprivation, relationship problems, family structure, unemployment, etc.

CHAPTER 7

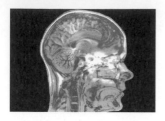

Treatment

Like psychiatric aetiology, psychiatric treatments are divided into *physical* — drugs and electroconvulsive therapy (ECT), *psychological* — the psychotherapies, and *social* interventions. A combination of approaches is usually used. Sometimes *compulsory* treatment is given.

Figure 7.1 gives a chronology of the major treatments currently in use.

Evidence-based treatment

For some psychiatric treatments there is good evidence of effectiveness, for others there isn't. We have searched the Cochrane Library (March 1998) for systematic reviews and have summarised the findings with * or ** in the text, the number of asterisks reflecting the confidence with which the conclusion is drawn. Absence of asterisks doesn't mean the treatment isn't effective, just that 'Cochrane evidence' is not available, in which case we have used standard sources of information and personal judgement to make our treatment recommendations.

• See the Appendix for more details on evidence-based psychiatry.

7.1 Drug treatments (psychopharmacology)

7.1.1 Introductory points

Drugs used in psychiatry fall into five categories (Table 7.1).

Consult a larger text for complete information about individual drugs, doses, side-effects and contraindications.

Certain principles govern the prescription of all psychiatric drugs (Table 7.2).

7.1.2 Antidepressants

Antidepressants are the first-line treatment for depressive disorders. They are effective**. The major classes are tricyclic antidepressants (TCAs) and selective serotonin reuptake inhibitors (SSRIs).

Tricyclic antidepressants (TCAs)

Not all drugs in this class are actually tricyclic in structure, but the collective term is used for all.

• *Mode of action.* Enhance noradrenergic and/or serotonergic (5-HT) function, by blocking presynaptic reuptake of the transmitters.

• *Uses.* Main use is in *depressive disorders*. 60–70% of patients respond. Less effective in very mild or very severe cases. Also reasonably effective in *neuroses*. Other uses include the treatment of *insomnia*, *chronic pain* and *nocturnal enuresis*.

• *Practical usage for depression.* Take 10–14 days to raise mood, although sedative and anxiolytic actions occur more rapidly. Side-effects are immediate, so build up dose gradually over 7–10 days. Can be given at night or in divided doses. After recovery, continue at full dose for at least 6 months then stop gradually.

HISTORY OF PSYCHIATRIC TREATMENTS

	Physical therapies	Psychotherapies
1900s		Psychoanalysis
1930s	Psychosurgery Electroconvulsive therapy (ECT)	Group therapy
1950s	Antipsychotics Monoamine oxidase inhibitors (MAOIs) Tricylic antidepressants (TCAs)	Brief psychodynamic therapy
1960s	Benzodiazepines	Family therapy Behavioural therapy
1970s	Lithium	Cognitive therapy
1980s	Selective serotonin reuptake inhibitors (SSRIs)	Cognitive behaviour therapy (CBT)
1990s	Atypical antipsychotics	

Fig. 7.1 When current psychiatric treatments entered regular use.

• *Side-effects.* Anticholinergic effects: dry mouth, blurred vision, urinary retention, constipation, tachycardia, delirium. Also postural hypotension, sexual dysfunction, weight gain, seizures.
• *Overdose.* Tachyarrythmias, convulsions, coma, death.

• *Cautions and contraindications.* Avoid in glaucoma, prostatism, recent myocardial infarction, cardiac failure, porphyria. Caution in epilepsy. Avoid with MAOIs. Alcohol in moderation. Drowsiness may impair ability to drive.

Which TCA to use?
The choice of which TCA to recommend depends mainly on:
• the desire for sedation;

Table 7.1 Drug treatments in psychiatry.

Class (synonyms)	Examples	Main indications
Antidepressants		Depression, neuroses
Tricyclics	Amitriptyline	
SSRIs	Fluoxetine	
MAOIs	Phenelzine	
Other	Venlafaxine	
Mood stabilizers	Lithium	Bipolar disorder
Anxiolytics (minor tranquillizers)		Anxiety, insomnia
Benzodiazepines	Diazepam	
Antipsychotics (major tranquillizers, neuroleptics)		Schizophrenia
Phenothiazines	Chlorpromazine	
Atypical	Clozapine	
Stimulants	Methylphenidate	Hyperkinetic syndrome

Table 7.2 Practical issues in psychopharmacology.

Principle	Example or consequence
Give the right dose	Antidepressant doses often too small, antipsychotic doses too high
Give the drug for the right amount of time	Antidepressants given too briefly, anxiolytics given for too long
Efficacy of each drug in a class is usually similar	Choice of drug determined by side-effects, toxicity and cost
Avoid combinations of drugs from the same class	No evidence for greater response rate, merely more side-effects
Non-adherence is a major reason for non-response Many patients don't believe in the drugs, only in the side-effects Antidepressants and antipsychotics are not addictive	Education and a good therapeutic relationship
Drugs are better than placebo but not always by much	Appropriate humility and awareness of alternative strategies

• tolerance of anticholinergic side-effects; and
• risk of overdose.

The properties of selected TCAs are given in Table 7.3. Our own favourite 'middle-of-the-road' TCA is lofepramine. It is as effective as other TCAs** and generally well tolerated.

Selective serotonin reuptake inhibitors (SSRIs)

The efficacy of TCAs and SSRIs in depression is similar**, but SSRIs have different and often fewer side-effects. They are much safer in overdose.

• *Mode of action.* Enhance 5-HT functioning by inhibiting the presynaptic 5-HT transporter.

• *Uses.* Main indication is depressive disorder. 60–70% response rate. Also used in mixed anxiety–depression, panic disorder, obsessive–compulsive disorder, bulimia nervosa, personality disorder and premenstrual syndrome.

• *Practical usage.* Like TCAs in terms of onset of action and duration of treatment. Fluoxe-

Table 7.3 Comparison of four usefully different tricyclic antidepressants (TCAs).

	Antidepressant dose (mg/day)	Sedation	Anticholinergic side-effects	Toxicity in overdose	Comments
Amitriptyline	75–250	+++	+++	+++	
Lofepramine	140–280	+	++	+	Dothiepin is similar
Clomipramine	75–250	++	+++	+++	? More effective than other TCAs in severe cases
Trazodone	150–600	++++	+	+	Fewer cardiac contraindications

tine, paroxetine and sertraline are widely used. Their properties are similar. Fluoxetine dose is 20 mg/day at breakfast.
• *Side-effects*. Usually well tolerated, though 15% of patients have nausea, abdominal discomfort, diarrhoea, insomnia, sexual dysfunction (anorgasmia) or agitation. No sedative or anticholinergic effects. No evidence that SSRIs cause suicide** or aggressive behaviour, despite media concerns.
• *Overdose*. Few effects. Rarely, if ever, fatal.
• *Cautions and contraindications*. Epilepsy. Avoid MAOIs; caution with lithium.

TCA or SSRI for depression?
A controversial question. SSRIs are now more commonly prescribed than TCAs because of their favourable side-effect and safety profile. However, the efficacy evidence (especially in more severe depression) and cost-effectiveness together (just) favour TCAs, *unless* there is:
• a serious suicide risk;
• intolerance of TCA side-effects; or
• a contraindication to TCAs.
If any of these apply, use an SSRI.

Monoamine oxidase inhibitors (MAOIs)
MAOIs such as *phenelzine* are second-line antidepressants. They are less effective than TCAs and potentially toxic. However, they have an important niche and are making a comeback with the development of the safer moclobemide.
• *Mode of action*. Prevent breakdown of noradrenaline, 5-HT and dopamine in synaptic terminals by the enzyme MAO. MAOIs are not addictive, though some have amphetamine-like metabolites.
• *Uses*. Main indication is in *atypical depression* (depression with phobic anxiety and hypersomnia;) or in depression not responding to TCAs or SSRIs.
• *Practical usage*. Ensure patient is aware of dietary restrictions and drug interactions (see below). Wait 2 weeks after stopping a TCA and 5 weeks after an SSRI. Give in divided doses.

• *Side-effects*. Postural hypotension, insomnia, ankle oedema, dry mouth, dizziness, agitation, headache.
• *Overdose*. Hypertension, delirium, coma, death.
• *Cautions and contraindications*. Prescribe with caution. MAO also metabolizes tyramine, so eating tyramine whilst on MAOIs (except moclobemide) can cause a hypertensive crisis (*'the cheese reaction'*) — headache, palpitations, fever, convulsions, coma. Certain food and drinks must be avoided, e.g. cheese, red wine, broad beans, pickled herrings, game, Marmite. Also dangerous interactions with many drugs including opiates, insulin, cold remedies, antiepileptics, SSRIs and some TCAs. An *'MAOI card'* should be carried. Avoid in cardiac or hepatic failure, and porphyria.
• *Choice of MAOI*. Moclobemide (300–600 mg/day). It is virtually free of the cheese reaction.

Other antidepressants
• Venlafaxine, reboxetine and mirtazapine are new antidepressants claimed to be at least as effective as SSRIs and/or to have fewer side-effects. Their clinical roles are not yet clear.
• In treatment-resistant depression, a variety of drugs are used to *augment* the action of TCAs or SSRIs (p. 89). These include lithium, tri-iodothyronine, L-tryptophan and pindolol.

7.1.3 Mood stabilizers
Mood stabilizers prevent mood swings in bipolar disorder. The main drug used is lithium.

Lithium
• *Mode of action*. Unknown. Possibly acts on neuronal second messenger systems.
• *Uses*. Main indication is prophylaxis of bipolar disorder. Also effective in acute mania (though antipsychotics work faster) and as an adjunctive treatment for depression. Sometimes used to treat behavioural disturbance in mental handicap.
• *Side-effects*. At therapeutic levels: fine tremor, metallic taste, dry mouth, thirst, mild polyuria, nausea, weight gain. Hypothyroidism

in 20% of women, rarer in men. Renal impairment may occur after prolonged use, but rare if toxic levels have been avoided.
• *Overdose*. Toxic symptoms occur above 2.5 mmol/l: coarse tremor, agitation, twitching, thirst, polyuria. Above 4 mmol/l: polyuric renal failure, seizures, coma and death. Toxic levels can occur in even mild dehydration, or on low salt diets — hence need for education and monitoring. Fatalities after overdose are not uncommon; survivors may be left with renal failure or brain damage.
• *Practical usage*. Explain dangers and how to avoid them. Do physical examination and investigations: electrolytes, creatinine clearance, thyroid function and ECG. During treatment measure lithium levels regularly (weekly at first, 3 monthly once stable). Dose (usually 400–1200 mg/day) is titrated to keep plasma levels at 0.5–0.8 mmol/l. Test thyroid and renal function every 6 months. Withdraw gradually.
• *Cautions and contraindications*. Many. Do not start if adherence likely to be variable or short lived. Avoid in renal failure, pregnancy. Avoid diuretics, angiotensin-converting enzyme inhibitors, high-dose antipsychotics. Caution with anti-inflammatory drugs, anaesthetics.

Carbamazepine
Carbamazepine, an anticonvulsant, is an alternative mood stabilizer if lithium is contraindicated or not tolerated. It is more effective than lithium in 'rapid cyclers' (p. 87).
• *Mode of action*. Unknown.
• *Practical usage*. Start at low dose (200 mg bd) and build up to 600 mg bd. Measure plasma levels if evidence of toxicity (ataxia, confusion, blurred vision). Check white cell count after a week.
• *Side-effects*. Erythematous rash or leucopenia — stop drug. Nausea, dizziness, drowsiness, hyponatraemia.
• *Cautions and contraindications*. Potent enzyme inducer, so other drugs metabolized faster — e.g. oral contraceptive. Avoid MAOIs. Avoid in hepatic failure, arrythmias, pregnancy.
Sodium valproate is also being used as a mood stabilizer and anti-manic drug.

7.1.4 Anxiolytics
Also known as *hypnotics* and *sedatives* if being used to help sleep. Benzodiazepines are the main class and in the 1960s and 1970s were very widely prescribed. With increased awareness about their dependency and withdrawal problems, SSRIs or TCAs have become the usual drugs for anxiety disorders. However, anxiolytics are still useful for short-term use.

Benzodiazepines
The former popularity of benzodiazepines is understandable: they are highly effective and free of unpleasant side-effects.
• *Mode of action*. Potentiate inhibitory transmission via the benzodiazepine binding site of the $GABA_A$ receptor. Genuinely addictive in some people.
• *Psychiatric uses*. Relief of *acute anxiety* and treatment of *panic disorder* or *phobic anxiety* and *insomnia*. Also used for *delirium tremens*, and to augment antipsychotics for sedation in *acute psychosis*.
• *Practical usage*. Diazepam (2–5 mg tds) is the standard anxiolytic. If intramuscular or intravenous administration may be needed, use lorazepam (1–4 mg qds). Temazepam (20 mg) is shorter acting and used for insomnia. In the USA, alprazolam (250 μg tds) is widely used for panic disorder.
• *Side-effects*. Drowsiness, 'hangover effects', headache, nausea, ataxia, dysarthria and cognitive impairment (due to sedation). Occasionally, disinhibition or aggression. Should not normally be prescribed for longer than 4 weeks, to prevent dependency. *Withdrawal symptoms*: rebound anxiety, insomnia, visual and auditory hallucinations, seizures. Manage by switching from short-acting benzodiazepines to diazepam, and taper dose over several weeks. As withdrawal is difficult and the drugs don't seem to cause significant harm, an alternative option in long-term users is to maintain them on the smallest achievable dose.
• *Overdose*: Rarely, if ever, fatal in healthy people. Flumazenil can be used to reverse effects.

- *Cautions and contraindications.* Caution with alcohol, driving.

Other anxiolytics and hypnotics
- Propranolol reduces the somatic symptoms of anxiety (tachycardia, tremor). Avoid in asthmatics.
- Buspirone is a non-sedating anxiolytic. Said not to be addictive. Takes several days to work.
- Chloral hydrate is a hypnotic used in the elderly.
- Zolpidem and zopiclone are newer hypnotics, claimed to produce fewer hangover effects and less tolerance than benzodiazepines.
- Low-dose tricyclic antidepressants also have anxiolytic and hypnotic effects — e.g. amitriptyline or trazodone.

7.1.5 Antipsychotics
Antipsychotics (*neuroleptics, major tranquilizers*) such as chlorpromazine and haloperidol are the mainstay of treatment for schizophrenia and other psychoses. Most antipsychotics have similar properties. There are also newer 'atypical' antipsychotics which have different side-effects, pharmacologies and perhaps effectiveness, than the conventional ('typical') ones.

Conventional antipsychotics
- *Mode of action.* Antipsychotic effects due to dopamine D_2 receptor antagonism and blockade of dopaminergic transmission in mesolimbic pathways. Not addictive.
- *Uses. Acute psychosis,* including acute schizophrenia and mania. Effective — 75% significantly better at 6 weeks (compared to 25% on placebo). Also effective in the *prevention of relapse in schizophrenia and other psychoses.* Other uses: delirium, psychotic symptoms in dementia and severe depression, and for sedation of disturbed or violent patients.
- *Practical usage.* Antipsychotic effects take 7–14 days to occur, though sedation occurs within hours. The use of very high doses (above recommended limits) for nonresponders is no longer acceptable — there is no evidence of greater efficacy and good

evidence of harm**. Antipsychotics can be given by intramuscular or intravenous injection for acute sedation, or in a depot preparation.
- *Side-effects.* Many: described below.
- *Overdose.* Arrythmias, hypotension, hypothermia, convulsions, coma, death.
- *Cautions and contraindications.* Glaucoma, prostatism, phaeochromocytoma, myasthenia gravis. Avoid high doses if on lithium. Can increase level of other drugs via hepatic enzyme inhibition.

Side-effects of typical antipsychotics
The first category are *extrapyramidal* side-effects (EPS), motor abnormalities related to the dopaminergic blockade in the basal ganglia. There are four types of EPS:
- *Acute dystonia* — painful contractions of muscles in the neck, jaw or eyes. Young men given high doses are vulnerable. Onset within hours or days. Treat with intramuscular or intravenous anticholinergics.
- *Parkinsonism* — decreased facial movements, shuffling gait, stiffness, sometimes tremor. Common in early weeks of treatment; manage by reducing dose or adding an anticholinergic (p. 65). Can be mistaken for depression or for negative symptoms in schizophrenia.
- *Akathisia* — feeling of restlessness, need to walk around. Very unpleasant. Occurs in first months of treatment. May be mistaken for psychotic behaviour. Treat by lowering dose and giving propranolol.
- *Tardive dyskinesia* — uncontrollable grimacing movements of face, tongue or upper body. Distressing and disabling. Occurs in 20% taking antipsychotics for 2 years. No way of predicting who will develop it. No reliable treatment, though reducing or stopping antipsychotic often helps. Vitamin E is ineffective**.

The miscellaneous collection of other side-effects is summarized in Table 7.4.

Which typical antipsychotic to use?
Typical antipsychotics differ in their chemical structure (a common exam question), potency and side-effect profile (Table 7.5), but not in efficacy — so the main factor affecting choice of

Table 7.4 Non-extrapyramidal side-effects of typical antipsychotics.

Side effects	Comments
Common side-effects	
Dry mouth	Due to anticholinergic effects (like TCAs). Tend to be inversely related to extrapyramidal side-effects
Constipation	
Blurred vision	
Urinary retention	
Sedation	Antihistaminic effects
Weight gain	
Postural hypotension	Blockade of α_2-adrenergic receptors
Amenorrhoea, galactorrhoea	Blockade of hypothalamic dopamine receptors
Inhibited erection and ejaculation	
Photosensitivity	Especially chlorpromazine
Rare but serious side-effects	
Neuroleptic malignant syndrome	Pyrexia, stiffness, autonomic instability, seizures, coma. Fatal in 20%. Stop antipsychotics temporarily if fever develops without clear cause
Seizures	
Tachyarrhythmias	
Retinal pigmentation	
Agranulocytosis	
Cholestatic jaundice	Especially chlorpromazine
Hypothermia	

Table 7.5 Comparison of some usefully different typical antipsychotics.

Structural class	Example	Dose range (mg/day)	Side-effects			
			Sedative	Extrapyramidal	Anticholinergic	Postural hypotension
Phenothiazine						
Aminoalkyl-	Chlorpromazine	25–800	++	+	++	+++
Piperidine-	Thioridazine	25–800	+++	+	+++	+++
Piperazine-	Trifluoperazine	5–50	++	+++	+	+
Butyrophenone	Haloperidol	1–20	+	+++	+	+
Substituted benzamide	Sulpiride	200–2400	+	+	+	+
Diphenylbutyl piperidine	Pimozide†	2–20	+	+++	+	+

† Pimozide has the advantage of a once-daily dose, but requires a pretreatment ECG.

drug is the side-effect profile — e.g. degree of sedation.

Depot antipsychotics

To improve treatment adherence in chronic schizophrenia, antipsychotics are often given as an intramuscular *depot injection* every 2–4 weeks. Common 'depots' are flupenthixol decanoate (mildly alerting) and fluphenazine decanoate (sedating).

Atypical antipsychotics

Clozapine is the key 'atypical' antipsychotic:
• it does not produce EPS;
• it is effective in 30% of schizophrenics who are resistant to, or intolerant of, typical antipsychotics;
• it may improve negative symptoms (p. 115), though the evidence is weak; and
• it works in a different way (perhaps via $5-HT_{2A}$ or dopamine D_4 receptors).

However, clozapine has problems:
• Agranulocytosis. Rare, but means the drug is given on a named patient basis and weekly white cell counts are mandatory.
• Weight gain, hypersalivation and sedation are common.
• Seizures at high doses.
• Very expensive (~ £3000 per year in the UK) — though cost–benefit analyses are favourable as inpatient care is reduced.

Clozapine is reserved for patients with schizophrenia who have not responded to, or are intolerant of, two other antipsychotics. Its use is also limited to those who will take daily medication (there's no depot) and have regular blood tests.
• Other new antipsychotics such as risperidone, olanzapine and quetiapine share some of the advantages of clozapine (especially the lack of EPS) and do not need blood tests.

Typical or atypical antipsychotics?

The clinical indications for atypical antipsychotics are still unclear. Our opinion is that first-line treatment of psychosis should still be with a drug from Table 7.5. If response is inadequate or side-effects troublesome, try olanzapine or risperidone, holding clozapine in reserve.

7.1.6 Anticholinergics

These drugs have no therapeutic value. They are used to counteract EPS of antipsychotics.
• Mode of action. Block muscarinic receptors. Their use may seem paradoxical given that other side-effects are attributed to the same action (Table 7.4). The rationale is that basal ganglia function depends on a dopaminergic–cholinergic balance; the EPS result from a relative deficiency of dopaminergic tone, so blocking cholinergic receptors brings them back into balance.
• Uses. Relief of dystonia and parkinsonism due to antipsychotics.
• Practical usage. Procyclidine (10 mg bd). It is also given parenterally to reverse acute dystonias.
• Side-effects. Can produce or exacerbate psychosis ('atropine psychosis') with confusion and visual hallucinations. Also memory impairment, euphoria. Anticholinergic side-effects of the antipsychotic itself may be worsened.
• Cautions and contraindications. Prophylactic and long-term use, though common, should be avoided for three reasons.

(a) Beneficial effects of antipsychotics are already maximal at a dose below that at which the EPS occur; antipsychotic dose reduction is therefore the logical response to these side-effects.

(b) Anticholinergics may increase the risk of tardive dyskinesia.

(c) Anticholinergics cause a 'buzz'. Patients may get addicted to them or sell them.

7.1.7 Prescribing in specific patient groups

Psychiatric prescribing in pregnancy, breast-feeding mothers, children and the elderly needs particular care. In general:
• choose a well-established drug;
• consult the British National Formulary;
• review the need for, and contraindications to, every drug;
• ensure patient (or carer) is aware of possible side-effects;
• monitor closely; and
• if in doubt, stop drug and review.

Pregnancy

Need to strike a balance between the wish to avoid all drugs for the sake of the fetus, and the maternal (and fetal?) morbidity of untreated psychiatric disorder.
• Antidepressants. TCAs and SSRIs (and ECT) not contraindicated. Dose requirement

increases in third trimester. Use of TCA at term may result in 'twitchy' baby.
• *Mood stabilizers*. Avoid carbamazepine. Lithium in the first trimester associated with small risk of cardiac malformations, and near term may result in neonatal hypothyroidism.
• *Anxiolytics and hypnotics*. Avoid.
• *Antipsychotics*. EPS in baby if taken near term.

Breastfeeding
Most drugs are excreted into breast milk. Weigh up need for medication vs. wish to breast feed.
• *Antidepressants*. TCAs (especially amitriptyline, imipramine) all right. SSRIs and MAOIs not recommended.
• *Mood stabilizers*. Monitor infant carefully if lithium used. Carbamazepine fine.
• *Anxiolytics and hypnotics*. Avoid benzodiazepines — can cause lethargy and failure to thrive.
• *Antipsychotics*. Can sedate infant (especially sulpiride). Not recommended.

Children
Child psychiatrists rather than GPs should prescribe. See Chapter 16.

The elderly
Prescribe at lower doses or increased intervals to compensate for slower metabolism and excretion. Always consider medication as a cause of delirium (p. 132).
• *Antidepressants*. TCAs may cause delirium (due to anticholinergic effects) and falls (due to postural hypotension). SSRIs are better if sedation not needed.
• *Mood stabilizers*. Not contraindicated.
• *Antipsychotics*. Use with caution in dementia — unexplained increased mortality.
• *Anxiolytics and hypnotics*. Notorious for causing delirium and falls. Avoid.

7.2 Other physical treatments

7.2.1 Electroconvulsive therapy (ECT)
An effective and safe treatment for severe depression. Its bad press reflects understand-able fears, misinformation and its past history of being given recklessly, without anaesthetic, to the wrong patients.
• *Mode of action*. Unknown. Causes many neurochemical and other changes in the brain.
• *Clinical indications*. ECT is mainly used, and with best evidence**, for *psychotic depression* including *depressive stupor* (p. 84), when response is often dramatic. Also used for *puerperal psychosis*, other forms of depression unresponsive to other treatments, and treatment-resistant *mania*.
• *Practical usage*. Get informed consent or use the Mental Health Act (p. 74), and perform a physical examination, ECG and routine blood tests. During a brief general anaesthetic with muscle relaxant, an electric current (~300 mC) is passed across the head to produce a generalized seizure lasting 30–60 seconds. Treatment can be either bilateral, with one electrode on each temple, or unilateral into the non-dominant hemisphere. Bilateral ECT is slightly more effective* but causes more short-term memory impairment. ECT is given twice a week for 6–12 treatments. A good response is predicted by a greater severity of depression (including psychotic and somatic symptoms), and a past response to ECT.
• *Side-effects*. Nausea and dry mouth from the anaesthetic. Headaches and memory loss for the hours surrounding the seizure. Significant long-term memory loss rarely, if ever, occurs — such complaints usually reflect continuing depression. However, there can be subtle deficits in recall of personal memories. No neuropathological effects have been found, even after hundreds of treatments.
• *Cautions and contraindications*. Anaesthetic contraindications. Avoid if suspected intracranial lesion (as intracranial pressure rises during seizure). ECT can be given in conjunction with TCAs and antipsychotics. Mortality rate is 5/100 000 treatments (which, especially in the elderly, is less than that seen with TCAs — and probably less than that for untreated depressive disorder).

7.2.2 Psychosurgery
In the 1940s and 1950s — prior to antidepress-

ants and antipsychotics—thousands of patients each year were operated on (without evidence of efficacy) to sever pathways between frontal lobes and limbic structures. Psychosurgery is still used occasionally for intractable obsessive–compulsive and depressive disorders, but only after wide consultations under the Mental Health Act and never without informed consent. Stereotactic procedures avoid most of the earlier complications (haemorrhage, seizures, death).

• Recent case series suggest worthwhile improvement in a third of cases — at the expense of some frontal lobe impairment and continuing ethical concerns. Results of randomized trials are awaited.

7.3 Psychological treatments (the psychotherapies)

7.3.1 Introductory points

All medical treatments take place in the context of a therapeutic relationship between doctor and patient. In psychotherapy, these factors are the currency of treatment itself.

The term psychotherapy used to refer to *psychodynamic* psychotherapy, which developed from Freudian origins (p. 54). Now, the term also includes *behavioural therapy* and *cognitive therapy,* which have a different source and rationale and which are becoming the standard form of psychological treatment because they are briefer and more convincingly effective.

There are three stages to understanding the various psychotherapies:
• the features common to all of them;
• the features which distinguish psychodynamic from newer psychotherapies; and
• the features of each specific psychotherapy.

Features common to all psychotherapies

• The therapist is appropriately trained, is empathic and interested, and listens and talks.
• Structure and boundaries are set (e.g. time, place, content of sessions).

• The therapeutic effect takes time.
• A therapeutic relationship is formed.
• A rationale is given.
• There is improvement of morale.
• Emotional arousal is involved — the person must engage in therapy enough to be aroused by it.

Features distinguishing psychodynamic from newer psychotherapies

The multitude of psychotherapies can by and large be put into one of two classes: either they are variants of psychodynamic psychotherapy; or they are based upon behavioural and cognitive theories (Table 7.6).

• The latter are sometimes called *manualized* therapies as they follow specific, written procedures.

7.3.2 Behavioural therapy

Behavioural therapy arose from the behavioural theories of experimental psychology (p. 53). The central idea is that adaptive behaviours can be learned and maladaptive behaviours unlearned. In turn, good behaviour leads to good feelings. Behavioural treatments are used in anxiety disorders and in mental retardation.

Exposure treatments

Exposure is a central component of behavioural treatment. Either the patient is reintroduced to a situation or behaviour he has come to avoid (e.g. an agoraphobic leaving the house), or he learns to stop an inappropriate excessive response (e.g. recurrent handwashing in obsessive–compulsive disorder).

• Exposure is usually graded (*graded exposure*). Sudden exposure (*flooding*)—such as shutting a claustrophobic in a lift until the panic subsides — also works, but is too unpleasant for routine use.

The elements of graded exposure are:
• The therapist characterizes the problem behaviour, its antecedents and consequences. He explains the nature of the treatment and its rationale.
• A step-by-step programme is developed with the patient's involvement. Homework tasks are

Table 7.6 Comparison of the two major classes of psychotherapy.

	Psychodynamic psychotherapies	Newer (manualized) therapies
Examples	Psychoanalysis Psychodynamic therapy	Behavioural therapy Cognitive therapy
Focus	Unconscious phenomena	Observable phenomena and behaviour
Temporal focus	The past (as evidenced in the present)	The present
Aim	Insight, self-understanding, and thence altered patterns of interpersonal behaviour	Direct, practice-driven change in behaviour and/or cognitions
Practical issues	Therapist listens and interprets Sessions unstructured	Therapist explains Sessions highly structured
Therapist	Extensive training (years) Usually psychiatrists	Briefer training (months) Psychologists, psychiatrists, nurse practitioners
	Key is therapist's skills and attributes	Key is therapist's adherence to treatment manual
Duration	Unspecified, can be prolonged (years)	Predetermined number of sessions (e.g. 12 weeks)
Efficacy	Unknown	Proven for several therapies and disorders
Main indications	Difficulties with relating Some personality disorders	Depressive disorder Neuroses Eating disorders

set which re-expose the patient to the situation to a degree which produces a tolerable level of anxiety which then subsides. In this way the patient is *desensitized* to the stimulus.

• Subsequent sessions review progress and problems and set the next series of tasks.

Mr Q had not been out of his house for 2 years, fearful he might faint in the street. His therapist elicited a detailed account of the problem, how it started, and its effect on Mr Q. She explained what behavioural treatment was and expressed optimism. They agreed a plan for Mr Q to do a task he felt he could just manage: to walk into his front garden and stand there briefly. He felt anxious doing so, but achieved this goal several times in homework sessions. He moved to the next steps: remaining there longer, then walking increasing distances. He was able to do the shopping, which reinforced his feeling of success. During the agreed 12 sessions he made steady progress which was maintained thereafter.

Other behavioural treatments

Many other treatments and techniques are based on the premise that changing behaviour and other bodily functions, such as muscular tone and posture, helps mental well-being. They include *relaxation training, assertiveness training, biofeedback* and *social skills training*. They are available in occupational therapy and physiotherapy departments, from private therapists and from self-help manuals.

7.3.3 Cognitive therapy

Cognitive therapy is based on cognitive and information processing theories (p. 54). The aim is to correct abnormal or unhelpful ways of thinking in order to improve mood and reduce anxiety. The main components of cognitive therapy are listed below:

• A detailed description of the problem is obtained. Particular attention is paid to identifying the thoughts (cognitions) and interpretations which have generated or are exacerbating the problem.

• The therapist formulates the problem in a way which makes sense to the patient.

• The patient is taught to challenge the negative and inaccurate ways of thinking which are maintaining the problem, and to practise thinking in more accurate and appropriate ways.

• Therapeutic techniques include education about the role of cognitions and their consequences, confirming the occurrence of particular thoughts and inferences using diaries, and simulation of events during the session. The patients are encouraged to do 'experiments' to test their beliefs.

• The same techniques are to be activated when negative thoughts reappear (*self-monitoring*).

Ms R had a depressive disorder. Her therapist helped her identify a number of negative thoughts such as: 'Nobody likes me'; 'I won't do things as I keep making mistakes'; and 'There's no point trying to change anything, it won't help'. The therapist formulated the depression as being maintained by the effect of this thinking on her mood and behaviour. He helped Ms R become aware of the distorted and negative slant of her thoughts and explained their possible origins and self-defeating consequences. They role-played alternatives and she practised challenging the thoughts and replacing them with positive ones. She became skilled at doing this. Her depressive thoughts and symptoms improved. At follow-up a year later she remained well, and was using the techniques whenever she felt negative cognitions or low mood creeping back.

Cognitive behavioural therapy (CBT)

In practice, cognitive and behavioural treatments are usually combined as *cognitive behavioural therapy* (CBT). In phobic anxiety, for example, this would involve both graded exposure to and intervention aimed at the underlying thoughts and beliefs. There is evidence for the efficacy of CBT (with varying proportions of C and B) in several disorders.

• In mild to moderate *depressive disorder*, CBT is at least as effective as antidepressants**.

• In *panic disorder* and *phobic anxiety*, CBT is probably the most effective treatment. Benefits are more persistent than with benzodiazepines, and avoid the problems of the latter. Also useful in other neuroses, including *chronic fatigue* syndrome and *obsessive–compulsive disorder*.

• In bulimia nervosa.

7.3.4 Psychodynamic psychotherapy

Following the arrival of the psychotherapies outlined above, psychodynamic psychotherapy has a limited role. Nevertheless, it remains important to know about its principles and its contemporary indications, and those of its concepts which remain useful.

Principles of psychodynamic psychotherapy

• Emotional and interpersonal problems result from *unconscious* processes, driven by psychological mechanisms and internal representations (of people and things) developed earlier in life.

• These processes can be revealed and resolved by gaining access to the unconscious mind. The therapist can do this in various ways (e.g. free association, hypnosis and dream analysis).

• The therapist is particularly interested in the patient's pattern of relationships, evidenced most directly by the patient's interactions with him.

• The therapist makes *interpretations* and draws connections between events and feelings.

• During therapy, the patient *gains insight* into his emotions and behaviour. The therapeutic effect may emerge directly from the self-understanding, and may be promoted (reinforced) by experimentation with new patterns of behaviour and relating which arise from it.

Psychodynamic concepts useful elsewhere

• *Transference*. The feelings and attitudes

patients develop towards their therapist. They represent emotions transferred to the therapist from the person to whom they were originally attached (usually a parent). Consider transference during any doctor–patient relationship if a patient starts to behave in an unexpected or unusual way (e.g. displaying inappropriate signs of affection, or threatening self-harm if an extra appointment is not given).

• *Countertransference*. The feelings a patient produces in the therapist (e.g. excessive involvement, attraction or dislike). Countertransference is influenced by the therapist's past experiences and relationships, but also gives clues to unconscious processes in the patient. More generally, it is valuable in that doctors need to be aware of the emotions evoked by patients, in order to try and understand their origins and ensure they do not affect their ability to treat the patient effectively.

• Defence mechanisms (see p. 55).

Contemporary indications for psychodynamic psychotherapy

It is now used mainly for 'personality difficulties', especially long-standing problems with relationships. Psychodynamic therapy also has a role in chronic neuroses and depressive disorders resistant to standard treatments. It

Fig. 7.2 Links between the major psychotherapies.

should be avoided in paranoid or dissocial personality disorder and psychosis.

• *Brief psychodynamic psychotherapy* compresses a psychodyamically oriented therapy to a feasible 10–20 sessions. The therapist takes a more active role and focuses on particular issues. There is evidence of moderate efficacy in depressive disorders.

7.3.5 Other psychotherapies
Hybrid therapies

The distinction between the two types of therapy in Table 7.6 is becoming blurred by hybrid psychotherapies which combine elements of both (Fig. 7.2):

• *Interpersonal therapy* (IPT) uses cognitive, behavioural and psychodynamic concepts and techniques to focus on the patient's relationships and the problems arising from them. It is of similar efficacy to CBT in depression and possibly superior in bulimia nervosa.

• *Cognitive analytical therapy* uses a cognitive approach to analyse earlier events and their influence on current feelings and behaviours.

Group therapy

Many psychotherapies have been adapted to treat several people at once. *Group therapy* originated from the belief that it is therapeutic to share experiences and feelings and to examine the relationships which form in a group.

• A *therapeutic community* is a form of psychodynamic group therapy where the participants are resident for 6–12 months.

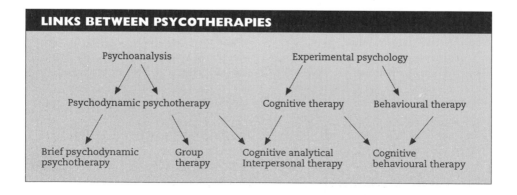

LINKS BETWEEN PSYCOTHERAPIES

Psychoanalysis

Experimental psychology

Psychodynamic psychotherapy

Cognitive therapy   Behavioural therapy

Brief psychodynamic psychotherapy

Group therapy

Cognitive analytical Interpersonal therapy

Cognitive behavioural therapy

Family therapy

Family therapy is based upon the view that the problem is located in the family rather than in the patient. The family 'system' is therefore the therapeutic target. Psychodynamic, behavioural and other concepts are used.

7.3.6 Informal psychotherapies

In addition to the 'formal' psychotherapies described above, *informal psychotherapies* are important too. They merge imperceptibly into the therapeutic component of all doctor–patient relationships.

• *Counselling* is a loosely defined activity whereby people are helped to cope with, or overcome, problems in their life. The counsellor serves as a support, a facilitator of emotional expression and a source of information, and as someone off whom ideas can be bounced. Counselling is provided in many non-psychiatric settings (e.g. Table 8.2).

• *Problem-solving therapy* is a structured mix of counselling and CBT. It improves well-being by helping the patient learn to deal with life's problems — by listing and specifying them, selecting an option for tackling each one, trying out solutions, and reviewing the effect. It is effective in mild neurotic and depressive disorders and is designed to be given by GPs and nurse practitioners in primary care.

• *Supportive psychotherapy* describes the supportive element of a therapist–patient relationship. All health-care workers — as well as relatives and friends — provide supportive psychotherapy whether they realize it or not. It does not aim to produce change, but to help people cope with adversity or insoluble problems over a sustained period—in part by maintenance of a sense of hope and a focus on achievable goals, however modest.

7.3.7 Practical issues in psychotherapy

Successful psychotherapy requires attention to several practical issues.

• *Select the right psychotherapy for the right patient.* Take account of the features predictive of good outcome to psychological treatment

in general: being motivated, articulate, able to tolerate emotional arousal, successful in some areas of life, as well as the specific indications and contraindications for each psychotherapy.

• *Prepare the patient for therapy.* Most people have either no idea, or the wrong idea, of what psychotherapy involves. Discussion about what to expect in therapy helps avoid inappropriate referrals and weeds out those unlikely to stay the distance.

• *Ensure the therapy is available.* Many psychotherapies are of limited availability or have a long waiting list. During this time, the referring doctor should offer continuing support or use the time for a trial of medication.

7.4 Social treatments

Social factors have major roles in the aetiology and maintenance of psychiatric disorders (p. 50), hence the need to ask about them in the psychiatric assessment (p. 13). Social factors also determine the environment in which therapy is given and affect its likelihood of success. Equally, social treatments — intervening to change some aspect of the person's circumstances — are themselves important therapeutic interventions.

• The need to attend to social factors and to integrate them with the medical aspects of psychiatric treatment was one motivation behind the development of community care (p. 80).

7.4.1 Acute social interventions

• *Psychiatric admission* is a major social intervention. It may relieve a crisis at home which is exacerbating the psychiatric disorder, or represent the best means of ensuring a homeless person gets a decent assessment.

• *Crisis intervention* also involves practical things like finding temporary accommodation, helping get emergency benefits or providing daily home visits.

7.4.2 Social interventions during psychiatric care

Practical social interventions are needed at some stage in most patients' care.

• Accommodation and financial problems are common. Help with rehousing requests, rescheduling debts, etc., is therapeutic by reducing stressors maintaining the disorder. Involvement of the patient in these processes can itself be therapeutic by giving them a sense of mastery over circumstances (which may have been perceived as overwhelming) and improving their practical social skills. These principles are built upon in problem-solving therapy.

• *Support and education* of the family and significant others is also an important part of the overall social package of care, even if specific family therapy is not being carried out.

• Isolation is a problem for many psychiatric patients. This can be addressed by home visits, arranging attendance at day centres, putting the person in touch with self-help groups, etc.

• In chronic psychiatric disorder, social and occuptional skills and self-confidence are often severely damaged. *Rehabilitation* involves continuing support of the kinds outlined above, as well as more extensive interventions such as the provision of sheltered accommodation and sheltered employment.

7.4.3 The wider social environment

Preventing domestic violence, child abuse and unemployment would no doubt improve the psychological well-being of the population. Whilst such utopian goals are not relevant for the management of individual patients, there are measures which can affect the prevalence or impact of such social ills:

• *Public education.* For example, the recent 'Defeat Depression' campaign of the Royal Colleges of Psychiatrists and General Practitioners was aimed at increasing public and medical awareness of depression and decreasing its stigma. Similarly, children can be taught the dangers of drugs.

• *Social policy.* Political decisions alter the social fabric and influence behaviours associated with psychiatric disorder. For example, taxation affects alcohol consumption and legislation determines health professionals'

response to suspected child sexual abuse. Some events are, however, beyond political control — e.g. the effect of national soccer results on deliberate self-harm rates.

7.5 Compulsory treatment

The nature of psychiatric disorder is such that some people refuse help, even though to do so puts their own health or that of others at risk. Therefore, psychiatrists sometimes treat people against their will.

• There is continuing debate about balancing the benefits of treatment against infringement of civil liberties, reflected in changes to mental health legislation from time to time.

7.5.1 Common law

Treatment without informed consent is technically an assault. However, in an emergency, a doctor may treat a patient without consent if rapid action is called for to save life — e.g. to maintain an airway in a comatose patient or to sedate an uncontrollably delirious patient. Such actions are carried out under the 'common law'.

• The limits of what can and should be done under common law are governed by the principle of doing what the public would consider reasonable (including acting where failing to act would be considered unreasonable). When in doubt, take advice from a senior colleague or your defence organization.

7.5.2 The Mental Health Act 1983

Apart from the specific sorts of emergencies mentioned above, compulsory treatment in England and Wales is carried out under sections of the 1983 Mental Health Act ('the Act') (Table 7.7).

• GPs are involved in most sections. All hospital doctors need to know about section 5(2).

• The Act only covers treatments for psychiatric disorder. It cannot be used if a patient refuses treatment for a medical problem—such as a stomach washout after an overdose, or to set a fracture — even if the patient is detained

Table 7.7 Key Mental Health Act sections and their uses.

Situation	Section
Psychiatric admission needed, for assessment	2
Psychiatric admission needed, for treatment	3
Psychiatric admission needed, psychiatrist not available	4
Stopping an inpatient leaving a hospital	5(2)
To allow police to find and take person to a safe place	135
To allow police to take person from public place to safe place	136
Psychiatric assessment or treatment of person on remand	35 and 36
Psychiatric treatment of convicted person	37 and 41

under the Act because of his psychiatric disorder.

Principles underlying the Act

• The person must have refused voluntary treatment.
• The person must be at risk of self-harm, self-neglect or harming others.
• The person's behaviour must be the result of a known or suspected psychiatric disorder. Disruptive behaviour, intoxication, drug abuse, etc., are not of themselves grounds for detention.
• For sections lasting a month or less, a loose definition of psychiatric disorder is adopted. For the longer-lasting sections, one of the following categories must apply: *mental illness* (not actually defined in the Act); *psychopathic disorder* (p. 148); or *mental impairment* (*mental retardation*).
• Implementation of most sections involves an *application* from an approved social worker (ASW) or the nearest relative, and a *medical recommendation* from a psychiatrist (consultant or senior registrar, approved under *section 12* of the Act). (Next-of-kin are rarely called upon to make an application because of the difficult position it puts them in.)
• Detained patients can appeal to hospital managers or to a Mental Health Review tribunal for the section to be discharged. A section is discharged anyway by the responsible psychiatrist once the patient's mental state no longer justifies it, and/or when he adheres consistently to treatment.

Section 2: Admission for assessment

• *Uses*: assessment of suspected psychiatric disorder, where admission is needed to prevent harm to self or others. It would apply, for example, to a man who set fire to his car because he believed it was possessed, or to a depressed lady who has tried to kill herself. Drug treatment can be given without consent, but use section 3 once treatment becomes the main reason for inpatient care.
• *Applied for by*: ASW, in consultation with nearest relative. Medical recommendation from a psychiatrist and another doctor (usually the GP; not a second psychiatrist from the same hospital—the two opinions are supposed to be independent). The ASW must have seen the person within the past 14 days, the doctors within 5 days.
• *Duration*: 28 days.
• *Right of appeal*: within first 14 days.

Section 3: Admission for treatment

• *Uses*: for treatment of severe, persistent psychiatric disorder (as described above) where admission is intended to improve the condition or prevent deterioration. Most patients on a section 3 have chronic schizophrenia. Some patients stay on a 'rolling' section 3 for years.
• *Applied for by*: as for section 2. Cannot normally proceed if the nearest relative objects.
• *Duration*: 6 months, renewable for 6 months then annually. Section 3 patients can go on leave for up to a month on a *section 17*. Before discharge, a *section 117* meeting is held to

discuss future management; there are statutory responsibilities for subsequent care (p. 81).
• *Right of appeal*: one appeal per 6 months. Reviews are instituted anyway if no appeal is made.

Section 4: Admission in an emergency
• *Uses*: for compulsory admission when a psychiatrist is not available and delay would be dangerous. Section 4 must not be used just because it is easier to organize than a section 2.
• *Applied for by*: ASW or nearest relative. Medical recommendation by any doctor, usually the GP.
• *Duration*: 72 hours, during which time a full assessment for a section 2 or 3 is made. No right of appeal.

Section 5(2): Emergency detention of an inpatient
• *Uses*: a '5–2' prevents a patient leaving *any* hospital where to do so would put their health in jeopardy. For example, a patient who is confused post-operatively and tries to run off, dripstand in tow, can be stopped at first under common law, but if he persists in attempting to leave, a section 5(2) should be used. A section 5(2) does not allow treatment to be enforced. (Section 5(4) can be used by psychiatric nurses to detain a psychiatric inpatient for 6 hours if no psychiatrist is to hand.)
• *Applied for by*: the responsible consultant or a named deputy. In a general hospital, this means the medical team managing the patient — a psychiatrist can't be called in to 'do the section'.
• *Duration*: 72 hours. During that time, a full Mental Health Act assessment must be carried out. Once completed, the section 5 is converted to a section 2 or 3 or it lapses. There is no right of appeal.

Other sections
• *Section 135* allows the police to enter private property and take a person to a place of safety (usually a hospital). The application is made by an ASW and granted by a magistrate. It lasts for 72 hours.
• *Section 136* is used if the police suspect that someone behaving dangerously or bizarrely in a public place has a psychiatric disorder. The police are empowered to take the person to a safe place (police station, casualty department or psychiatric hospital). It lasts for 72 hours.
• *Sections 35–38* are used by a court to send a remanded or convicted offender to a hospital for psychiatric assessment or treatment. *Section 47* allows for the transfer of someone from prison to hospital.
• ECT may not be given without consent to detained patients, except the first treatment in an emergency. A second opinion must be obtained and *section 58* used before the course of ECT proceeds.

The Mental Health Act in Scotland
Compulsory treatment is covered by the 1984 Mental Health Act (Scotland). The principles are similar to those described above, but the section numbers and some practical details are different (Table 7.8).

7.5.3 Other aspects of the law and psychiatry
All psychiatrists find themselves involved with the law from time to time. . . . Though not all the issues are strictly related to treatment, they are summarized here for convenience.
• *The law and child psychiatry*. Children under 16 are subject to different laws and conventions. The main legislation is the Children Act (1989). Consult a child psychiatric team or social services for advice.
• *Writing court reports*. Psychiatrists are often asked to write a report on behalf of a patient who has been charged with an offence. Usually they are asked to give an opinion as to whether psychiatric factors contributed to the offence, or how it should be dealt with. Forensic psychiatrists have specialist expertise and deal with the more serious crimes (p. 79).
• *Compensation claims*. Psychiatrists may be asked to support a patient's claim for compensation, where a psychiatric disorder is

Table 7.8 Key Mental Health Act sections in Scotland.

Situation	Section	Features
Admission for assessment	24	Lasts 72 hours. Recommendation by a doctor plus social worker or a relative
To prolong assessment of patient on section 24	26	Lasts 28 days. Requires second medical recommendation
Admission for treatment	18	Lasts 6 months, renewable. Recommendations from two doctors, one specially approved, plus support of social worker or a relative. Also needs sheriff's approval

alleged to have been caused by a particular event, such as post-traumatic stress disorder after an accident.

• *Fitness to make a will or enter into contracts.* Psychiatric opinion may be sought regarding a person's competence to make a will, get married, sign a hire purchase agreement, and so on.

• *Fitness to drive.* Psychiatric disorders and medications can impair driving by affecting judgement or concentration. Psychiatrists should warn patients of this and of their duty to inform the relevant authority if in doubt. A person may not drive for 6 months after a psychotic episode. People with dementia (even mild cases) have an excess of accidents and should be discouraged from driving.

• *Medical confidentiality.* There are exceptional circumstances which over-ride the principle of medical confidentiality in psychiatry. For example, if a patient tells you he is planning to murder his wife (perhaps because he has a delusion that she is a devil), you should warn her. If unsure what to do, seek advice.

7.6 SUMMARY: KEY POINTS

• Psychiatric disorders are treated with drugs (psychopharmacology) and psychological methods (psychotherapy). Social interventions are important too.

• The main classes of drugs are antidepressants (tricyclics and SSRIs), antipsychotics, anxiolytics and mood stabilizers.

• The main psychological treatments are cognitive behavioural therapy and psychodynamic therapy.

• The choice of treatment in a particular case depends upon:
  diagnosis;
  predominant symptoms;
  personality (e.g. suitability for psychotherapy);
  patient's preference; and
  availability.

• There is good evidence for the efficacy of most drug treatments, but they do have limitations and side-effects. Cognitive behavioural therapy is of proven benefit for several disorders.

• For each treatment, think of:
  what type it is;
  how it may work;
  which disorder(s) it is used for;
  how it is given;
  how effective it is, if known; and
  its side-effects and contraindications.

• A minority of patients are treated without their consent under the Mental Health Act.

CHAPTER 8

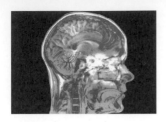

Psychiatric Services

8.1 The who and where of psychiatry

This chapter covers the organization of psychiatric services and the personnel involved — issues important in understanding how psychiatric treatments are delivered.

8.1.1 Multidisciplinary teams

Most psychiatrists work in *multidisciplinary teams* as one amongst several mental health professionals. The psychiatrist's particular role generally centres on:
* making diagnoses;
* prescribing medication; and
* taking medicolegal responsibility.

The other members of multidisciplinary teams usually include the following:
* *Psychiatric nurses.* In the community they are called *CPNs (community psychiatric nurses).* CPNs perform much of the day-to-day work of the *community mental health team* (CMHT). CPNs are often the *key worker* (see below); they perform many of the assessments, and they give medication. Some have additional therapeutic skills (e.g. in cognitive therapy) and are called *nurse practitioners.*
* *Clinical psychologist.* Many teams have a clinical psychologist, who provides psychological assessments and treatments.
* Social services departments have statutory responsibilities affecting psychiatric patients which the team *social workers* fulfil. For example, the social worker takes the lead role in assessing social circumstances and arranging accommodation, helping with benefits, etc. ASWs *(approved social workers)* have a key role in Mental Health Act applications (p. 73).
* *Secretary/administrator.* Teams generate a lot of paperwork and its members are out and about. A person at the team base who takes messages, arranges meetings and manages the office is therefore a key figure.
* *Other team members* may include occupational therapists, accommodation officers, befrienders, etc.

8.1.2 Where psychiatry happens

Traditionally, psychiatry was based in mental hospitals and most patients were inpatients. Over the past 30 years, psychiatric services have progressively moved to other settings (Table 8.1).

The shift of psychiatry to the community has occurred for several reasons:
* The community is where psychiatric disorders present and their context lies.
* Public preference and social attitudes.
* Long-term inpatient care is rarely necessary and sometimes harmful.
* Economic and political pressures.

Despite these trends, inpatient care remains an important component of psychiatry for:
* Assessment of suspected severe psychiatric disorder.
* Those at significant risk of suicide.

• Those dangerous to others as a result of psychiatric disorder.
• Treatment of acute schizophrenia, mania and severe depression.
• Longer-term care of some patients with dementia, chronic schizophrenia and mental retardation.

As the number of psychiatric hospital beds has fallen, the threshold for admission has risen and an increasing percentage of inpatients are psychotic, disturbed and detained. This is especially true in inner cities, and has stimulated efforts to ease the pressure. Research suggests that admission could be avoided in up to 40% of cases using day hospitals or community 'crisis teams'. At present these alternatives are not widely available.

Voluntary organizations
Voluntary organizations and self-help groups are important additional sources of support and help for many people, including those not receiving formal psychiatric care. A selection are listed in Table 8.2.

Table 8.1 Where psychiatry happens.

Psychiatric hospital
Inpatient wards
Outpatient clinic
Day hospital
Special hospitals
General hospital
In casualty
Medical clinics and wards
Psychiatric beds
Primary care
By GP
By psychiatrist
Community
Mental health centre
Domiciliary visits
Penal system
Police station
Prison
Private sector

8.2 Psychiatric subspecialties

The major branches of psychiatry are delineated by the patients' age and/or type of disorder:
• General adult psychiatry.
• Psychogeriatrics (psychiatry of old age).
• Child and adolescent psychiatry.
• Liaison psychiatry (psychological medicine).
• Substance abuse.
• Forensic psychiatry. The interface of psychiatry with the law.
• Mental retardation (learning disabilities). See Chapter 17.

8.2.1 General adult psychiatry
Adults with psychiatric disorders are looked after by general adult psychiatrists unless their problems come into the domain of another

Table 8.2 Voluntary organizations relevant to psychiatry in Britain.

Alcoholics Anonymous and Al-Anon	[Local number]
Alzheimer's Disease Society	0171 360 0606
CarersLine (Carers' National Association)	0345 573369
Cruse (bereavement care)	0181 940 4818
Depression Alliance	0171 633 9929
DrinkLine (national alcohol helpline)	0345 320202
MIND (National Association for Mental Health)	0181 519 2122
Narcotics Anonymous	0171 351 6794
National Schizophrenia Fellowship	0181 974 6814
Relate (formerly Marriage Guidance)	0178 857 3241
Samaritans	0170 875 1111
SANE (Schizophrenia—A National Emergency)	0171 724 8000

subspecialty. The boundaries are blurred and depend on local factors. The division between adult and old-age psychiatry is particularly variable; it may be based purely on age, or on a combination of age and cognitive impairment.

• Since most of this book is concerned with general adult psychiatry, it is the features that distinguish the other subspecialties which are emphasized in the following sections.

8.2.2 Psychogeriatrics (old-age psychiatry)

• Old-age psychiatrists deal with all psychiatric disorders in the elderly and not just dementia.

• Concurrent physical problems and medications affect presentation and management. For example, constipation is common in the elderly and is therefore a less useful diagnostic sign for depression; it may also produce delirium; it may limit the dose of antidepressant which can be given.

• Psychogeriatric CMHTs have close ties with geriatrics and social services. This is necessary given the prevalence and nature of dementia, and the frequency of associated physical and social problems of elderly patients with psychiatric disorders.

The vignette illustrates how a common psychogeriatric scenario may evolve.

Mr A is 75 and has become forgetful. A domiciliary visit reveals cognitive impairment and depressive symptoms. He lives with his healthy wife. A trial of antidepressants does not help, and his dementia worsens. Routine investigations are negative and you diagnose probable Alzheimer's disease. An occupational therapist visits to assess his daily living skills. His wife can care for him with help from meals on wheels and visits from a CPN. You liaise with the GP regarding Mr A's leg ulcers (which make him delirious when infected); the GP prescribes antibiotics and a district nurse. Two years later Mr A is severely cognitively impaired and aggressive, seemingly in response to hallucinations. His wife is not coping. The psychologist gives advice about managing his behaviour, which settles on a small dose of an antipsychotic. You help his wife by organizing day care and a 2-week

respite admission for him. The next year she dies. No other relatives can care for Mr A. You admit him and look for a nursing home. A social worker sorts out the finances. Six months later Mr A breaks his hip. After discussion with his son, conservative management is agreed on. Mr A is kept comfortable in the nursing home and dies the next day.

8.2.3 Child psychiatry

Children's psychiatric problems differ in important respects from those of adults, and the approach to their assessment and management is also different (Chapter 16).

• A child psychiatrist requires a detailed understanding of physical and psychological development. Many are also trained in paediatrics.

• The first contact with child psychiatric services may come from the GP, paediatrician or school educational psychologist.

• A child psychiatry team includes specialized social workers, nurses and psychologists. Some of the team may concentrate upon family therapy.

• When inpatient care is needed, other family members may be admitted too, to help in evaluation.

8.2.4 Liaison psychiatry

Liaison means link, and liaison psychiatrists provide an important link between general psychiatric services and medical and surgical services. They are based in general hospitals and are principally concerned with three patient groups:

• People who present to casualty having self-harmed. Some hospitals have trained counsellors to carry out screening of all self-harm patients; elsewhere it is left to the medical or nursing staff to decide when to refer to a psychiatrist.

• General hospital patients, whose doctors suspect they have a psychiatric problem contributing to, arising from, or complicating, their medical disorder.

• Patients whose symptoms are medically unexplained (p. 172).

Liaison psychiatrists offer specialist opinions on these patient groups; they may then offer treatment themselves, or suggest referral to other local psychiatric services.

You are asked to see Mr B in casualty. He is 49 and has taken an overdose. He is not suicidal but does have depressive and anxiety symptoms. You suspect he has an adjustment reaction after recent life events.You offer him an appointment for the following week, give him a number to call if he feels the urge to self-harm again, and phone his GP. On review, the severity of depression becomes clearer. He starts antidepressants. You discuss the case with the local general adult CMHT who take over his care. Six months later you are called to see him on a surgical ward where he is awaiting a cholecystectomy. The houseman discovers his psychiatric history and wants your opinion on his mental state. Mr B is fine, but you note that his antidepressant, an MAOI (p. 61), interacts with analgesics. You advise discussion with the anaesthetist.

8.2.5 Substance misuse psychiatry
The workload of this specialty comprises:
• Management of psychiatric disorder resulting from alcohol or drug abuse.
• Management of the psychological and social consequences of substance misuse. Many people have complex and multiple needs which both cause and result from their substance misuse.
• Inpatient care for detoxification (in some units).
• Advice and support for people wanting to stop misusing drugs or alcohol.
• Advice to other doctors managing patients in whom substance misuse may be a factor.
• Public education about the dangers of substance misuse.

Counsellors and outreach workers play important roles in this specialty in addition to the CPNs and social workers. Considerable efforts are made to make contact with people with drug or alcohol problems who are unwilling to attend a medical setting. Co-operation with physicians is important because of the medical problems which often coexist.

Mr C had delirium tremens. After recovery, a liaison psychiatrist referred him to the drug and alcohol clinic. You take a history and discuss his medical condition with his GP. He is given information about alcohol and introduced to a CPN who will visit regularly to review progress and give support. A social worker investigates his benefit problems and contacts his ex-wife about access to his children. Mr C does not want medication to help him abstain. Things go well until he loses his job. He starts to drink heavily and drops out of care. He turns up later wanting admission for detoxification. Needle marks are noticed. He admits to injecting heroin and is found to be hepatitis B positive. He again cuts down his alcohol and denies taking other drugs thereafter. He gets a new job and his wife returns to him. He has had no relapse when seen a year later.

8.2.6 Forensic psychiatry
Forensic means 'of the courts'. All psychiatrists become involved in forensic issues for various reasons:
• Writing psychiatric court reports or attending court on behalf of a patient.
• Assessment of local offenders with suspected psychiatric disorder. Court diversion schemes are being developed to reduce the delay such people experience before receiving psychiatric help.
• A forensic history (e.g. of assault) may affect management decisions even if not directly related to current psychiatric problems.

Forensic psychiatrists become involved in the following circumstances:
• Psychiatric assessment of persons charged with serious crimes, especially murder.
• Providing treatment for convicted prisoners with a psychiatric disorder. This includes running psychiatric care in regional secure units and the Special Hospitals (e.g. Broadmoor).
• Giving advice to other psychiatrists encountering forensic issues. For example, in assessing dangerousness.

In practice, the decision as to when a patient with a forensic history should be transferred to the forensic psychiatric services depends on the crime, the likelihood of recurrence and the availability of resources.

8.3 Community psychiatric care

Logically, this term should refer to the management of all psychiatric problems outside hospital; numerically this would mainly comprise patients in primary care (p. 170). Usually, however, the term is limited to patients receiving long-term care from psychiatric services. Such patients have often had a psychiatric admission and formerly would either have remained in hospital or have attended as day patients or outpatients.

Most patients with psychiatric disorder can and should be managed in the community. However, making the move from hospital- to community-based care over the past 20 years has posed problems:

• Hospitals have closed before community services are fully in place.

• Community care is not a cheap option, and has been under-resourced.

• A considerable burden is placed upon relatives.

• It is difficult to provide care for the people often most at need—the homeless, those with complex psychiatric and social problems, and those whose illness interferes with treatment adherence.

Together, these factors have led to a gap between the intention and reality of community care. A separate influence has been the homicides committed by psychiatric patients. Though these are extremely rare, public concern has led to an emphasis upon the supervision of patients in the community and how this should be legally enforced.

8.3.1 Principles of community psychiatric care

• Psychiatric problems are managed at the patient's home, in GP surgeries or in local mental health centres. To facilitate this, the psychiatrists usually divide workload into geographical sectors.

• Care is provided by a multidisciplinary CMHT.

• Management includes social interventions as well as drug and psychological treatments.

• Admission is reserved for severe episodes and crises. Transitions between inpatient and community care should be as smooth as possible.

• Most patients are treated with their consent. A few need some form of legal coercion (see below).

8.3.2 Practicalities of community psychiatric care

There are various models of community care — and much jargon. The two main varieties are *case management* and *assertive community treatment* (ACT).

• Case management and ACT are not treatments, but ways of delivering treatment. For patients with psychosis, their main purpose is arguably to improve adherence with medication, since this is the major determinant of outcome.

Case management

An important feature of case management is that each patient has a *key worker* (also called a *case manager*). In CMHTs, the key worker is usually a CPN or a social worker. The key worker has responsibility for:

• assessing the patient's needs — psychiatric, medical and social—as well as risk assessment;

• identifying which person or agency is best placed to meet which need;

• drawing up a written *care plan*; and

• co-ordinating and reviewing the care plan.

In Britain, the specific form of case management by which community care is delivered is the *Care Programme Approach* (CPA).

• The CPA has been augmented by the introduction of *supervision orders* and a *supervision register*. The supervision order (also called *supervised discharge*) requires a patient to live at a specified address and attend for follow-up (but they cannot be forced to accept treatment). The *supervision register* is intended to be a list of all patients in psychiatric care thought to be at significant risk of self-harm, neglect or causing harm to others. Its use remains patchy and controversial because of concerns about medical confidentiality and civil liberties, and the practical problems of its use.

Ms D is 27 and has been admitted with schizophrenia. A CPN attends the ward round and discusses her future care with the CMHT. He agrees to be the key worker and the CPA is implemented. Ms D has been made homeless and unemployed, so the CPN liaises with the social worker and sorts out financial arrangements and accommodation in a group home. After discharge, he visits weekly, monitoring her mental state and giving Mrs D her depot. The psychiatrist sees Ms D every 6 months or whenever there is cause for concern. An exacerbation of her illness is managed at home with support and increased medication. The CPN begins therapy with Ms D's family, who are supportive but overinvolved. However, Ms D relapses and is found wandering the street in a state of neglect. She is detained under section 3 of the Mental Health Act. When she is almost ready for discharge, a section 117 meeting plans her future care.

Assertive community treatment
Recent evidence suggests that the CPA is not very effective, and there is now a shift towards ACT as the chosen form of community care. ACT differs from case management in that:
• It is more intensive. Each team member has fewer patients under their care but is more involved.
• The team meet more of the person's needs themselves (rather than involving other agencies).
• Responsibility for the patient's care is held collectively by the CMHT.
• It is highly focused on patients with severe psychiatric disorder (especially psychosis) who have a history of multiple admissions or failure to engage and remain in treatment.

There is some evidence that ACT may prevent admission and improve clinical outcome.

8.4 Groups with special psychiatric needs

Some groups are particularly likely to have their psychiatric needs unrecognized or unmet. Special efforts and creative solutions are needed to ensure that this does not happen.

8.4.1 The homeless
Difficulties
• Multiple social and medical needs.
• High prevalence of psychiatric disorder.
• Hard to engage and keep in treatment.

Solutions
• ACT.
• Outreach workers.
• Realistic goals.

8.4.2 Ethnic minorities
Difficulties
• Diagnoses harder to make because of cultural differences in presentation.
• Language barrier (especially for the mental state examination, where nuances of meaning are important).
• Concerns about racial prejudice and stigmatization.

Solutions
• Awareness of cultural differences in how psychiatric disorders present.
• Trained interpreters.
• Staff reflecting ethnic make-up of community.

8.4.3 People with comorbidity
Difficulties
• Worsens prognosis.
• Hampers management.
• Increases risk of violence (especially psychosis + personality disorder + substance misuse).

Solutions
- Recognition of comorbidity.
- Extra resources.
- Prioritize management plans — target major and soluble problems.

8.4.4 Medical patients
Difficulties
- Present with somatic complaints.
- Focus is on medical not psychiatric symptoms and interpretations.

Solutions
- Education of non-psychiatric doctors.
- Good liaison with psychiatry services.

8.4.5 Health-care workers
Difficulties
- Reluctance to admit to psychiatric problems.
- Increased risk of alcohol misuse and suicide.
- Hard to maintain confidentiality.
- Blurring of boundaries between being a colleague and a patient.

Solutions
- Confidential, publicized, accessible local arrangements.
- British Medical Association helpline (0645 200169) and National Counselling Service for Sick Doctors (0171 935 5982).

8.5 SUMMARY: KEY POINTS

- Psychiatric services are provided by multidisciplinary mental health teams, within which the psychiatrist works with psychiatric nurses, social workers and other disciplines.
- Each patient has a key worker.
- Most psychiatric patients are treated in the community. Community care in the UK is delivered through the care programme approach (CPA).

CHAPTER 9

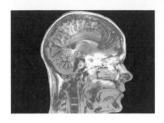

Mood Disorders

In mood disorders there is a persistent disturbance of mood beyond the fluctuations we all experience. Normal mood (*euthymia*) can become lowered (*depression*) or, less commonly, elevated (*mania*).
• The term depression may refer either to someone's current mood or to their underlying diagnosis (even if they aren't presently depressed).
• Mood is also called *affect*, hence the alternative term *affective disorders*.

9.1 Clinical features of mood disorders

Review the relevant parts of the core assessment (p. 9) and the mood module (p. 23).

9.1.1 Clinical features of depression

The most characteristic (though not invariable) symptom is *low mood*. It may be described as such, or as feeling 'down', 'fed up', 'tired', etc. In addition there are *psychological symptoms* (e.g. anhedonia) and sometimes *somatic symptoms* (also called *biological* or *vegetative*) such as weight loss.
• The pattern of symptoms, as well as the therapeutic and prognostic implications, differs according to the severity of the depressive episode (Table 9.1).

• Symptoms must have been present for at least 2 weeks.

Mild depression
Though the word 'mild' is used, the term is reserved for people who are more than just unhappy.
• Mild depression is the commonest form of depressive episode.
• Patients often complain of feeling stressed or tired. Anxiety symptoms (p. 98) frequently coexist, leading to the term *mixed anxiety–depression* (p. 96). Somatic symptoms are absent. Low mood may not be apparent to the interviewer. Suicidal thoughts can occur but serious self-harm is unusual.

Moderate depression
This is the 'textbook' form of depressive episode seen by psychiatrists (because it is the severity at which referral tends to occur).
  Mood is objectively as well as subjectively depressed (p. 11). Somatic symptoms are present (Table 9.1). The appearance is usually of *psychomotor retardation* (p. 23); however, others become *agitated*, seemingly unable to get peace from what's on their mind. Anhedonia (p. 23) is important and characteristic, leading the person to give up their normal pleasurable activities. It may be exacerbated by *poor concentration* and *lack of motivation*. Thoughts are negative and pessimistic, centring upon

Table 9.1 Symptoms of depression.

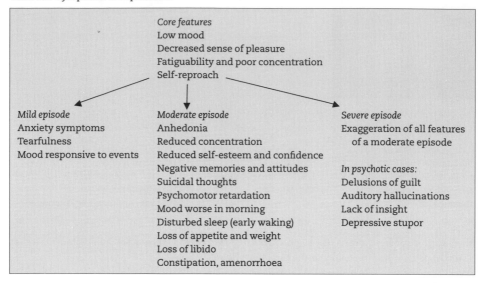

Core features
Low mood
Decreased sense of pleasure
Fatiguability and poor concentration
Self-reproach

Mild episode
Anxiety symptoms
Tearfulness
Mood responsive to events

Moderate episode
Anhedonia
Reduced concentration
Reduced self-esteem and confidence
Negative memories and attitudes
Suicidal thoughts
Psychomotor retardation
Mood worse in morning
Disturbed sleep (early waking)
Loss of appetite and weight
Loss of libido
Constipation, amenorrhoea

Severe episode
Exaggeration of all features
   of a moderate episode

In psychotic cases:
Delusions of guilt
Auditory hallucinations
Lack of insight
Depressive stupor

unpleasant memories, past failings and a bleak future.
• *Hopelessness* and *helplessness* readily supervene, not only reinforcing the depressed mood but leading to suicidal thoughts.

Severe and psychotic depression

In severe depression, the symptoms of a moderate depressive episode are magnified. A deep and pervasive sense of gloom is evident. The person no longer experiences nor is interested in the normal pleasures of life. There are many somatic symptoms.
• Suicidal thoughts and intentions become prominent.

Depression at its most severe becomes *psychotic depression* (also called *depressive psychosis*). Worries and perceived misdemeanours become delusional in intensity. The patient may believe she is dead or that part of her is (*Cotard's syndrome*); she may experience *auditory hallucinations* with voices cursing her or telling her she is worthless.
• Psychomotor retardation can increase to the point where the person sits motionless and

mute — *depressive stupor*. This used to end in death from dehydration; it now calls for emergency ECT.

9.1.2 How depression presents

Many depressed patients do not complain of, or admit to, low mood, but present because of the associated cognitive, behavioural or somatic symptoms (Table 9.2). Consequently, depression often surfaces in non-psychiatric settings (p. 172), and all doctors must be alert to the various guises of depression.
• Somatic presentations of depression are particularly common in Asian cultures.

9.1.3 Clinical features of mania

As with a depressive episode, there is a spectrum of severity: *hypomania* describes mild or moderate mood elevation; *mania* denotes the real McCoy (Table 9.3).

Hypomania

Hypomania is a happiness and zest for life in excess of that which is normal. *Concentration* is impaired and *distractibility* occurs. Thoughts flit

Table 9.2 Ways depression presents.

Example	Depressive explanation
An old man who's forgetful	Poor concentration
A mother unable to cope with her child	Lack of motivation and pleasure due to postnatal depression
A student with weight loss and fatigue	Depressive symptoms
A woman worrying about having AIDS	Obsessional ruminations secondary to depression
A man with panic attacks	Anxiety symptoms secondary to depression
Marital conflict	About sex, due to husband's depression and loss of libido
In casualty after failed hanging attempt	Depression is common in people with real suicidal intent

Table 9.3 Symptoms of mania.

Hypomania	Mania
Excessively happy, gregarious	Symptoms of hypomania magnified
Distractible and irritable	Grandiose delusions
Rapid, voluminous speech	Auditory hallucinations
Expansive ideas	Flight of ideas
Disinhibited behaviour	Pressure of speech
Increased energy, decreased sleep	Commission of inappropriate or dangerous acts
Partial insight preserved	Lack of insight

from one topic to another. Sleep is reduced and the night may be spent spring cleaning or writing a novel. Neither will be done well or completed. An *infectious gaiety* easily switches to *irritability*, in frustration that others do not share their enthusiasm.

• A degree of insight is retained and a daily routine just about maintained. However, hypomania often heralds the impending onset of mania.

Mania

The features of hypomania are exaggerated and psychotic symptoms emerge. Thought processes become disordered and jumpy (*flight of ideas*; p. 26), accompanied by *pressure of speech* (p. 25). Manics develop *grandiose delusions*, believing themselves blessed with special powers. They may hear voices supporting these beliefs. Unfortunately, reality and gravity

supervene, and people with mania do things they later regret. For example, they may be promiscuous or generate huge debts.

9.2 Types of mood disorder

9.2.1 Classification of mood disorder

Having identified that depression or mania is present, establish the type of mood disorder. The classification of mood disorder is confusing, but can be simplified using the categories shown in Fig. 9.1.

First consider the unlikely but important possibility that the mood disorder is attributable directly to an 'organic' (p. 126) cause — i.e. a medical disorder or a consequence of substance misuse. If so, the diagnosis is *organic mood disorder*. This category and its implications are discussed further on p. 133.

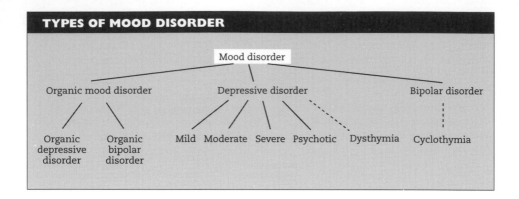

Fig. 9.1 Classification of mood disorders.

The vast majority of cases have no specific organic cause of this kind; any known organic factors are just one component of a multifactorial aetiology. In all these cases, the diagnostic decision is between *bipolar disorder* and *depressive disorder*, the latter sometimes prefaced with *unipolar* (Fig. 9.1). This distinction is

Fig. 9.2 Course of mood disorders.

based upon the presence or absence of a history of mania.

• Bipolar and depressive disorders are in turn subdivided according to *course* and *severity* (Fig. 9.2).

9.2.2 Depressive disorder

Depressive disorders are categorized according to the severity of the current episode into mild, moderate, severe or psychotic (Fig. 9.1). If there has been more than one episode the label *recurrent depressive disorder* is sometimes used (Fig. 9.2).

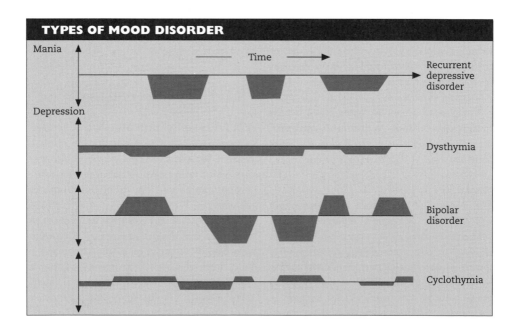

Dysthymia

Some people are rarely, if ever, free of depressive symptoms. The clinical picture is of long-standing low mood of insufficient severity for even mild depressive disorder. This is called *dysthymia*. It is experienced as a lack of pleasure in life and things being an effort.

Exacerbations supervene at times of stress.
• It is controversial whether dysthymia is the result of a 'depressive personality' or a chronic, mild form of depressive disorder. The latter view is supported by genetic evidence; it also encourages dysthymia to be seen as treatable, which to a degree it is.

9.2.3 Bipolar disorder

As with depressive disorder, ICD-10 distinguishes people who have only had one episode of mania (diagnosis: 'manic episode') from those who have had two episodes of mania and/or a depressive episode (diagnosis: 'bipolar disorder'). For example, a lady might have 'bipolar disorder, current episode manic'.

• The main feature of *bipolar disorder* is that normal mood is interspersed with depressive and manic episodes. The frequency and magnitude of the shifts is very variable, as is the proportion of depressive to manic mood swings, though sooner or later depression always occurs.
• 'Bipolar disorder' is synonymous with *manic depression* or *manic depressive psychosis*.
• 'Unipolar manic disorder' is not a category — since almost everyone with mania sooner or later becomes depressed and therefore bipolar.

Cyclothymia

Cyclothymia is mild, chronic bipolar disorder. Like dysthymia, it is sometimes viewed as a personality trait. Psychiatric help is rarely sought since the mild mood elevations are pleasant and associated with enhanced productivity and creativity.

Table 9.4 A glossary of mood disorder terms.

Atypical depression	Depression with increased sleep, appetite and phobic anxiety
Agitated depression	Depression with prominent anxiety, agitation, restlessness. Contrasted with *retarded depression*, a distinction of value when deciding which antidepressant to use
Bipolar I and II	Bipolar disorder where there has (bipolar I) or hasn't (bipolar II) been an episode of mania as opposed to hypomania
Brief recurrent depression	Depression severe enough to warrant a diagnosis of depressive disorder but which only lasts a few days and recurs frequently
Double depression	Depressive disorder on top of dysthymia
Endogenous depression	Depression attributed to genetic and biochemical factors. Prominent somatic symptoms, hence the term *biological depression* was formerly applied to similar cases
Melancholia	Depressive disorder with anhedonia and somatic symptoms
Mixed affective state	Simultaneous manic and depressive symptoms
Rapid cycling	Bipolar disorder with >4 episodes a year
Reactive depression	Depression as a response to external (c.f. endogenous) circumstances. Lacks somatic symptoms
Seasonal affective disorder	Depression which recurs in autumn or winter, associated with increased sleep and carbohydrate craving. May respond to bright light therapy

9.2.4 Other terminologies

We have already mentioned an array of labels applied to mood disorders. Unfortunately many more are also in use (Table 9.4).

9.3 Epidemiology of mood disorders

Table 9.5 shows figures from recent population surveys.

The finding of more depression in women than men is robust. Possible explanations include:
• genetic predisposition;
• hormonal influences;
• social pressures;
• greater willingness to admit to depressive symptoms; or
• the fact that depressed men are given other diagnoses, such as alcohol misuse.

Mood disorders are getting commoner. The reason is unknown.

Table 9.5 Occurrence of mood disorders.

	Bipolar disorder	Depressive disorder
Lifetime risk (%)	1	15
One-month prevalence (%)	0.4	5
Sex ratio	1:1	1:2
Mean age of onset	20s	Any

9.4 Management of mood disorders

9.4.1 Depressive disorders

Many depressed people do not consult a doctor and, if they do, the diagnosis may be missed. The first management principle is therefore better recognition of depression by sufferers and doctors.

• Psychiatrists see only a small percentage of people with depressive disorder, highlighting the need for GPs to be confident about its diagnosis and treatment (p. 170).

Once depression has been diagnosed, it must be treated appropriately. The first-line treatment is usually an antidepressant. Before prescribing, consider various issues which affect your decision (Table 9.6).

Drug treatment of depression

A depressive episode will respond to an antidepressant, either a tricyclic antidepressant (TCA) or selective serotonin reuptake inhibitor (SSRI), in over 60% of cases. The chances of success can be increased by simple procedures (Table 9.7; see also Table 7.2).

Mr S has a depressive disorder. He is married and unemployed. He had a similar episode 5 years ago which resolved without treatment after several months. He doesn't accept he's depressed and blames his problems on his own inadequacies. You explain that he has a depressive illness which needs treatment. You summarize what depression is and how antidepressants work, including their

Table 9.6 Factors affecting management decisions in depression.

Question	Implication/example
Is there a serious suicide risk?	May need admission. Use SSRI not TCA as less toxic in overdose
Are there psychotic symptoms?	Add an antipsychotic to the antidepressant, or use ECT
What are the predominant symptoms?	Affects choice of drug. For example, use sedative antidepressant if insomnia
Is there a past history of depression?	Use the treatment which worked last time
Is there a past history of mania?	Caution with antidepressants (may precipitate mania)
Are there medical problems?	Avoid tricyclics after recent myocardial infarction

Table 9.7 Prescribing antidepressants effectively.

Principle	Examples
Educate about antidepressants	Take 14 days to work. Side-effects get better. Non-addictive. Effective
Give an adequate dose	Amitriptyline at least 100 mg/day. Lofepramine 210 mg/day. Fluoxetine 20 mg/day
Check drug is being taken	Non-adherence is common reason for apparent non-response
Give the drug for long enough	Therapeutic trial should be 2 months, at adequate dose
Attend to the psychosocial aspects	Restore hope. Educate about depression. Practical advice

possible side-effects and delayed onset of action, but also emphasize that they will help him sleep and reduce his anxiety. You tell him to take 50 mg amitriptyline tonight, and increase to 150 mg/day over a week. His wife is present and agrees to supervise his tablets. You will see him in a week to review progress.

After recovery, continue treatment at the same dose for at least 6 months before tapering off the drug over several weeks. Explain that maintaining treatment in this way reduces the high risk of relapse in the months after a depressive episode. In people who do relapse, reinstitute the treatment which worked the first time, but continue it for longer. There is good evidence in favour of prolonged use of antidepressants in a prophylactic role, and none that long-term use is harmful.

Mr S adhered to treatment. His sleep and agitation improved rapidly. The depressive symptoms responded over the next few weeks, though it was necessary to increase amitriptyline to 200 mg/day for a full response. He became constipated but this improved with laxatives. He subsequently accepted that he had been ill, and conceptualized the amitriptyline as correcting a chemical imbalance thus helping him to solve life's problems more effectively. He no longer blamed himself for his redundancy, and found a new job. His wife confirmed the improvement. On your advice, he remained on medication for a further 6 months.

Non-response to first-line treatment

In a third of cases, depression does not respond to a first-line antidepressant (or to a psychological treatment). If there has been absent or poor response:

• Check the antidepressant has been taken as prescribed. Measuring plasma levels can be useful.

• Increase to the maximum tolerated and recommended dose.

• Review the case. Is the diagnosis right? Could there be powerful perpetuating factors, such as Cushing's syndrome, marital strife or alcohol misuse? Can their impact be reduced?

Having addressed these issues, there are various options. The commonest decisions are to switch from TCA to SSRI (or vice versa) or to try a second drug from the same class. There isn't much evidence in favour of either strategy. Alternative options are:

• Add lithium or tri-iodothyronine to the antidepressant if depression is severe. See lithium cautions (p. 61).

• Cognitive behavioural therapy (CBT), if available.

• Switch to a monoamine oxidase inhibitor, especially if there are phobic anxiety symptoms. See cautions (p. 61).

• Add an antipsychotic or try ECT if there are psychotic symptoms.

• Try one of the newer antidepressants (p. 61).

• Psychiatric referral, if not already made.

Psychiatric referral for depression

Unresponsive or problematic cases of depressive disorder warrant psychiatric referral:
• for a second opinion on diagnosis or treatment options;
• for specialist use of combinations of drugs or rarely used agents;
• for access to psychological services, occupational therapy, etc.; and
• for admission (e.g. because of suicide risk or need for ECT).

Psychological treatment of depression

Cognitive behavioural therapy (p. 69) and interpersonal psychotherapy (p. 70) are effective alternatives to antidepressants in mild and moderate depressive disorder. There is little evidence that combining an antidepressant with a psychological treatment is more effective than either alone.
• Psychological therapies are often preferred by patients, being seen as curing underlying problems rather than just treating symptoms, and they are attractive to practitioners because there is some evidence that they reduce the risk of relapse of depression. However, the shortage of trained therapists limits their use.

There are no good predictors of who will benefit from psychological rather than pharmacological treatment of depression. A few pointers are:
• depression not severe (as defined in Table 9.1);
• 'psychological mindedness';
• willingness to engage in therapy and carry out homework tasks; and
• preference for psychological treatment or reluctance to take medication.

9.4.2 Bipolar disorder

Treatment of mania

Mania usually requires admission, often compulsorily, and the patient may need to be restrained. A manic episode is best treated with antipsychotics (for the psychotic component) and benzodiazepines (for sedation). Lithium, ECT and sodium valproate are second-line treatments.

• If the patient is already on lithium, check the blood level to assess recent adherence.
• Untreated, mania can last for months. Death from 'manic exhaustion' was well recognized before treatments became available.

Treatment of depressive episodes in bipolar disorder

Depressive episodes in bipolar disorder are often severe. In addition to the use of antidepressants, they may require antipsychotics or lithium (partly because antidepressants used alone can precipitate mania). Admission and ECT may also be necessary.

Prophylaxis of bipolar disorder

Long-term lithium treatment reduces the risks of relapse in bipolar disorder, and treating bipolar disorder early may improve its outcome. Lithium should be offered to all those who have had two manic episodes, or one manic and one depressive episode. However, do not prescribe it unless both patient and doctor intend to continue it for at least 2 years—stopping it earlier carries a high risk of rebound mania.
• Counselling and various tests are needed before lithium is given (p. 61). Patient education may also increase adherence.
• In over a third of patients, lithium is either ineffective or not tolerated, or there are contraindications. Carbamazepine and sodium valproate are alternatives.
• Relapses in bipolar disorder are often heralded by non-specific symptoms (e.g. deteriorating sleep). Some patients become adept at recognizing and responding to these warning signs.

9.5 Prognosis of mood disorders

9.5.1 Depressive disorders

Over 50% of people with one depressive episode will have another. The more severe the depression, the worse the prognosis; most people with psychotic depression suffer

multiple episodes, and 10% never recover fully.
• Suicide occurs in one-in-eight people with recurrent depressive disorder.

9.5.2 Bipolar disorder

By its nature, bipolar disorder runs a remitting and relapsing course. The prognosis is worse in young-onset cases, rapid cyclers (Table 9.5), and women. The suicide risk is similar to that for depressive disorder.
• The disruption caused by the illness, especially the manic phases, often leads to problems in maintaining relationships, employment and accommodation.

9.6 Aetiology of mood disorders

9.6.1 Organic factors and mood disorders

As with all psychiatric disorders, the aetiology of mood disorders involves a mixture of biological, psychological and social factors (Chapter 6). There are, however, a few cases which are considered to be due directly and overwhelmingly to a specific medical or pharmacological cause, and ICD-10 groups these in a category of 'organic mood disorder', as mentioned on p. 133. Organic causes of mood disorder are summarized in Table 9.8.

A 65-year-old man presented to his GP with insomnia, anorexia, back pain and weight loss. He also felt fed up and irritable. The GP diagnosed depression with somatic symptoms. On referral, examination revealed bony tenderness over his lumbar spine and a hard nodular prostate. He was hypercalcaemic and anaemic. He had metastatic carcinoma of the prostate. His depressive symptoms resolved as his hypercalcaemia was treated.

• Clearcut cases of organic mood disorder are very rare, and even where the diagnosis is made, psychological and social factors are still likely to be relevant for its course and treatment. The category's value stems from the

Table 9.8 Organic causes of mood disorder.

Depression	Either	Mania
Endocrine and metabolic		
Cushing's disease		Hyperthyroidism
Addison's disease		
Hypothyroidism		
Hypercalcaemia		
Folate deficiency		
Neurological		
Cerebrovascular disease		
Epilepsy		
Multiple sclerosis		
Brain tumour		
Head injury		
Systemic lupus erythematosus		
Parkinson's disease		
Drug-associated		
Beta-blockers		Amphetamines
Digoxin		Steroids
Anti-epileptics		L-DOPA
Barbiturates		Antidepressants

occasional patient (as in this vignette) where depression is the presenting feature of a serious medical disorder, hence the need for psychiatrists to consider the possibility early in the diagnostic process—and do an appropriate physical examination (p. 14).

9.6.2 Aetiology of depressive disorders

Depression is the result of an interaction of genetic, social, psychological and biological factors (Table 9.9).
• There is a large genetic predispositon (heritability 40–50%). The same genes are involved in all types of depressive disorder (but not bipolar disorder) and overlap with those associated with anxiety disorders. The number and identity of the genes is unknown. They operate directly to increase risk of depression, and via effects on personality and social factors (Fig. 9.3).
• The major environmental factors are bad childhood experiences and current psychosocial adversity (p. 51).
• Depression is associated with the personality attributes of *neuroticism* (anxiety, obsession-

Table 9.9 Aetiology of depressive disorder.

Genes
Past experiences
  Emotional deprivation
  Parental separation
  Traumatic events
Psychosocial adversity
  Life events
  Lack of support
  Medical illness
Psychological factors
  Neuroticism
  Learned helplessness
  Negative cognitive style
Biological factors
  5-HT system abnormality
  HPA dysfunction

ality, poor coping with stress), low self-esteem and perhaps negative cognitive style (p. 53).
• The main neurochemical suspect is hypofunction of monoamine neurotransmitter systems (5-HT, noradrenaline) in conjunction with HPA axis dysfunction (p. 57).

Fig. 9.3 Pathways to depression.

• Lesions of the subcortical white matter are associated with late-onset depressive disorder.

9.6.3 Aetiology of bipolar disorder
• Bipolar disorder is strongly heritable. Monozygotic : dizygotic twin concordance is 75% : 25%. Relatives of someone with bipolar disorder have an increased incidence of both bipolar and unipolar depressive disorder. Loci on chromosomes 18 and X are implicated. There is some evidence for anticipation (p. 166) and maternal inheritance.
• No childhood risk factors are known. Life events can precipitate the initial episodes; once the disorder is established, its course is increasingly immune to environmental circumstances.
• Neurobiologically, instability in the monoamine systems is suspected.
• Always consider drug-induced mania (an example of organic mood disorder) in young people with no family history of bipolar disorder. In someone first presenting in middle age, exclude cerebrovascular disease, tumours and medication side-effects.

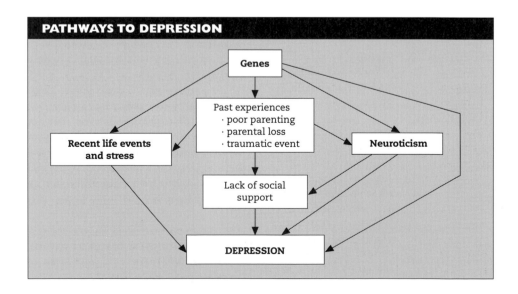

PATHWAYS TO DEPRESSION

Genes

Past experiences
· poor parenting
· parental loss
· traumatic event

Recent life events and stress

Neuroticism

Lack of social support

DEPRESSION

9.7 Other aspects of mood disorders

9.7.1 Puerperal disorders

The puerperium is a hormonally and psychologically turbulent time. It is traditional to group puerperal psychiatric disorders together, because their clinical picture and management differ somewhat from those of similar disorders occurring at other times.

Maternity blues

The 'blues' are a tearful, irritable, labile mood which affect over 50% of mothers on the third or fourth postnatal day. The symptoms resolve within days without treatment, though explanation and reassurance may be needed. There is no association with mood disorder.
• Maternity blues may be due to the precipitous fall in sex steroids after delivery as well as to the psychological impact of childbirth and concerns about mothering.

Postnatal depression

Postnatal depression tends to start within a month of delivery. Fifteen per cent of mothers are affected. The woman's worries may centre on her failings as a mother, on her baby's well-being, she may be fed up with his incessant demands.
• As well as the standard mood and risk assessments, ask about the mother–baby relationship. Postnatal depression can put the baby at short-term risk and, if untreated, may lead to persistent problems with bonding and child development.
• Most cases are managed at home. Use supportive measures, including explanation and reassurance to the mother and her family. Mobilize resources (e.g. the local mothers' group), and liaise with the GP, midwife, health visitor, etc. Many cases resolve within a few weeks, but antidepressants (cf. breastfeeding; p. 66) or psychological treatment should be considered if the disorder is moderate or severe. If admission is necessary, it should be to a mother-and-baby unit, in order to maintain and observe their relationship.
• Postnatal depression is commoner in women with a history of psychiatric disorder and in those lacking support. A postnatal change in sensitivity of the dopaminergic system is implicated.

Puerperal psychosis

Puerperal psychosis used to be due mainly to sepsis, i.e. it was an organic psychosis. Now, the typical picture is of a psychotic mood disorder or schizoaffective disorder (p. 123). About 1/500 women are affected. Onset is usually in the second postnatal week. Risk factors include a past or family history of psychosis and being a primigravida.
• The disorder can be severe. Perplexity and confusion are characteristic. The baby is at potential risk because of the mother's delusions or because she is so preoccupied by her symptoms that he is neglected. The assessment should specifically address these issues.
• Admission is usually necessary. Treatment is with antipsychotics and antidepressants, and with a low threshold for ECT — which generally produces a dramatic response. Recovery is usual, but there is a 25% relapse rate after the next delivery and a 50% lifetime risk of further psychosis.

9.7.2 Premenstrual syndrome

Up to 80% of women suffer from symptoms in the days before their period: irritability, depression, abdominal bloating and breast tenderness. However, a specific premenstrual syndrome has proved difficult to validate (and is not included in ICD-10).
• If a woman complains of premenstrual syndrome, establish the symptoms and their relationship to the menstrual cycle. Ask her to keep a diary — it may transpire that the symptoms are present at other times in the cycle too.
• There is some evidence for the efficacy of SSRIs, oestrogens, gonadotrophin agonists, danazol and CBT. There is no good evidence for progestogens or primrose oil.

9.7.3 Other psychiatric issues specific to women

Abortion, sterilization, hysterectomy and the menopause have all been said to cause psychiatric distress, especially mood and anxiety disorders. There is no good evidence for any of these claims. (Though psychiatric morbidity is high in women undergoing hysterectomy, it falls postoperatively.) Each of these events may, however, act as a stressor relevant to the understanding or treatment of a disorder occurring soon afterwards.

9.7.4 Grief

If you know you are dying, or you have been bereaved, emotional pain and turmoil are to be expected. Many of the features overlap with those of depression. Psychiatrists and other doctors are asked to assess or support people during these times, so it is necessary to know:
• the characteristic psychological reactions to impending death and to bereavement; and
• the features which distinguish these from depressive disorder.

Normal grief

People may grieve a death (bereavement) or other major loss, or may grieve an impending event (anticipatory grief). The responses are forms of adjustment reaction. Three stages of grief have been described.
• *Shock and disbelief.* On being told of the event there is an initial numbness which usually lasts a day or two. It is a form of stress reaction (p. 100). Behaviour may be acutely disturbed.

• *Preoccupation and 'depression'.* This central phase involves a preoccupation with the deceased. In the early stages anger is common, directed at doctors, God or other target of blame. Uncontrollable crying, low mood, social withdrawal and somatic symptoms akin to those of depression may be pronounced. The voice or image of the deceased may be vividly perceived, though usually with an 'as if' quality rather than being truly hallucinatory.
• *Acceptance and resolution.* With time, the person comes to terms with the event, symptoms subside and life begins to return to normal. This phase may take several months to start, and several more to be completed. Recurrence of grief is common around anniversaries.

In uncomplicated grief, counselling and support (e.g. from Cruse) may be useful. Such grief should not be labelled as a disorder but viewed as a natural though painful process. The therapist should, however, be on the look-out for signs of abnormal grief or depressive disorder.

Abnormal (pathological) grief

Grief can be abnormal in three ways:
• *Absent or delayed grief.* There may be no outward signs of grief despite an event of grief-inducing proportions (absent grief). Grief usually begins a few weeks later (delayed grief).
• *Prolonged grief.* An arbitrary term which tends to be used if there are prominent symptoms more than 6–12 months later. At this time, actively consider depressive disorder and

Table 9.10 A comparison of depression and grief.

	Depression	Grief
Suicidal thoughts	Common, driven by low mood	Transient, driven by wish to be with deceased
Blame for situation	Self	Other people or fate
Psychomotor retardation	Yes	No
Psychotic features	In severe cases. Mood congruent	No, though may imagine seeing or hearing deceased
Symptom course	Pervasive	Fluctuating

the need for counselling or specific treatments.
• *Excessive grief.* The intensity of grief is unusually great — this may reflect the person's closeness to the deceased, their personality or a depressive disorder.

Grief and depression
A depressive disorder occurs in a third of grieving people, and is severe in 20%. As the foregoing sections show, it is not easy to decide when the threshold from grief to depression is crossed. However, certain features help, apart from simply an excessive intensity or duration of the grief (Table 9.10).
• The person may need persuading that their suffering is not just the pain of normal grief but a depressive disorder needing treatment.

9.8 SUMMARY: KEY POINTS

• The central feature of mood disorder is excessively lowered or elevated mood.
• Psychological and physical symptoms are associated with altered mood. In depression, anhedonia, poor sleep and suicidal thoughts are common. In mania, look for increased energy, rapidity of thoughts and grandiosity.
• Depressive disorder results from an interaction of genes with bad childhood experiences, personality factors and current social adversity.
• Depression often goes undiagnosed, especially when it presents with physical symptoms in non-psychiatric settings. It is also undertreated.
• Suicidal risk needs detailed and regular assessment.
• Antidepressants are the usual first-line treatment. Give an adequate dose and continue for at least 6 months after recovery. CBT is as effective as antidepressants for mild and moderate depression but is not widely available. ECT is reserved for severe, resistant cases.
• Mania is treated acutely with antipsychotics and sedatives; lithium is used for prophylaxis in bipolar disorder.

CHAPTER 10

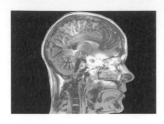

Neuroses

10.1 General characteristics of neurosis

We all experience anxieties and worries. Sometimes these emotions become excessive or inappropriate. *Neurosis* ('to do with the nerves') is the traditional term for these emotional disorders. Anxiety is the emotion most affected.

Although anxiety is central, neurosis often presents because of the associated cognitions (e.g. recurrent thoughts about illness), behaviour (e.g. the agoraphobic who cannot leave her house) or physical symptoms (e.g. palpitations). Neurosis is divided into a number of *neurotic disorders* (*neuroses*), according to the balance between these components and the focus of the symptoms.
• For an introduction to the clinical features of neurosis, review the module (p. 27).
• Neurosis is common and underdiagnosed in primary care and general hospitals (p. 170).
• Neuroses can be chronic and disabling — and are associated with twice the expected mortality rate.

10.1.1 Neurosis and neurotic symptoms
In someone presenting with neurotic symptoms, ask two questions:
Do the symptoms warrant any diagnosis?
• Assess whether symptoms are diagnostically significant, based upon their intensity, number and pervasiveness, and the resulting *dysfunction* — are they interfering with the person's life? If they are long-standing, could they be a personality trait or part of a personality disorder (Chapter 15)?
Are the symptoms part of another psychiatric disorder?
• Neurotic symptoms can occur in *any* psychiatric disorder, especially depression (see below), and in medical disorders (p. 172).
• Each of these disorders is diagnosed by the presence of their characteristic features. If present, they 'trump' neurosis in the diagnostic hierarchy (p. 4).

Assuming the diagnosis is one of neurosis, next decide which neurotic disorder is present (see below).

Neurosis and depression
Depressive symptoms are common in neurosis, and neurotic symptoms are common in depressive disorders. Indeed, in many patients seen in primary care, anxiety and depressive symptoms coexist in similar proportions. The diagnosis of *mixed anxiety–depression* is useful in such cases.

10.1.2 Epidemiology of neurosis
If mixed anxiety–depression is included, neurosis afflicts about 15% of the population at any one time (p. 170). Most of the neurotic

disorders are twice as common in women. The onset is generally between early adulthood and middle age, though children also suffer from similar disorders (p. 155).

10.1.3 Management of neurosis

The neuroses share a common responsiveness to certain drugs and psychological treatments.

• Antidepressants and anxiolytics are both effective, though anxiolytics are now less commonly used because of the risk of dependence. Antidepressants are effective in neurotic disorders, even those without a significant depressive component; they could also be called 'antineurotics'.

• Cognitive behavioural therapy (CBT) (p. 69) is as effective as medication. The specifics of treatment differ somewhat between the individual neuroses.

• Social interventions (e.g. removal of stressors) are part of management.

10.1.4 Prognosis of neurosis

In the community, the majority of neurotic disorders are acute and transient. Psychiatrists see primarily chronic and intractable cases. The usual good prognostic factors apply: no personality disorder; the patient is motivated to get better; short history.

10.1.5 Aetiology of neurosis

Neuroses have a multifactorial aetiology.

• Neuroses — and neuroticism (p. 92) — are moderately heritable. This genetic relationship may explain why neuroses are commoner in people with anxious cluster personality disorders (p. 147).

• Alterations in the 5-HT and noradrenergic systems probably mediate anxiety symptoms.

• Cognitive factors and behavioural conditioning (p. 53) are important psychological processes.

• Abnormal illness behaviour and the sick role (p. 52) are relevant sociological concepts.

These influences can be put together to make an aetiological model like that for mood disorder (p. 91), in which neurosis is a result of

Table 10.1 Neurotic disorders.

Anxiety disorders
  Phobic anxiety
  Panic disorder
  Generalized anxiety
Obsessive–compulsive disorder (OCD)
Reactions to stress
  Acute stress reaction
  Adjustment disorders
  Post-traumatic stress disorder
Dissociative disorders
Somatoform disorders
Neurasthenia
Depersonalization–derealization syndrome

stressors interacting with personality attributes and genetic predisposition.

10.1.6 The specific neuroses

The ICD-10 neurotic disorders are summarized in Table 10.1 and described in the following sections.

• We only mention the aetiology, prognosis or management of specific neuroses where there is something significant to add to that described for neurosis in general.

• *Mild* neuroses can rarely be placed into one of these categories. The term *undifferentiated neurosis* or *minor emotional disorder* is used instead.

• Variants of neurosis are seen in particular cultures. These include *amok* (dissociative disorder in Indonesia) and *koro* (severe anxiety about penis shrinkage in Chinese men).

10.2 Anxiety disorders

As the name suggests, these are neuroses dominated by *anxiety, anxious thoughts*, and the bodily *symptoms of sympathetic arousal* which accompany it (Table 10.2).

• The nature and prominence of the bodily symptoms (e.g. chest pain) often leads the patient to present initially to medical services.

Anxiety disorders are divided into three subtypes: *phobic anxiety, panic disorder* and *generalized anxiety* (Table 10.3).

10.2.1 Phobic anxiety

The anxiety is *situational*, restricted to the experience or anticipation of the phobic stimulus. There is avoidance of situations associated with the stimulus (e.g. a severe mouse phobic may avoid old houses or nature programmes). Although it produces immediate relief from anxiety, avoidance is counterproductive because it reinforces the phobia. Avoiding avoidance is a key part of behavioural treatments (p. 67).

• The differential diagnosis is from other anxiety disorders. Occasionally, phobic anxiety may arise from delusions. Phobia of disease (hypochondriasis) is classified separately (p. 102).

• Psychological treatment is based on graded exposure and desensitization — behavioural therapy (p. 67). A cognitive component may be added. Antidepressants and anxiolytics are also effective.

Agoraphobia

One of the commonest phobias is *agoraphobia* ('fear of the market place'). Intense anxiety is provoked either by open spaces, or large spaces which are crowded and difficult to escape from (e.g. supermarket queues). Panic attacks are common, so a diagnosis of *panic disorder with agoraphobia* is often made.

• The cognitions concern fear of fainting, dying or other catastrophe, rather than a fear of shops or spaces *per se*.

Table 10.2 Common symptoms of anxiety.

Component	Prominent features
Emotion/mood	Anxiety, irritability
Cognitions	Exaggerated worries and fears
Behaviour	Avoidance of feared situations, checking, seeking reassurance
Bodily (somatic)	Tight chest Shortness of breath (hyperventilation) Palpitations 'Butterflies' Tremor Tingling of fingers Aches and pains Poor sleep Frequent desire to pass urine and motions

Table 10.3 Features distinguishing the three types of anxiety disorder.

	Phobic anxiety	Panic disorder	Generalized anxiety
Occurrence of anxiety	Situational	Paroxysmal	Persistent
Associated behaviour	Avoidance	Escape	–
Associated cognitions	Fear of situation	Fear of symptoms	Fear of future (worry)

Table 10.4 Symptoms of agoraphobia.

Component	Prominent features
Emotion	Situational anxiety—in shops, crowded large places
Cognition	Thoughts of collapsing and being left helpless in public
Behaviour	Avoidance of panic-provoking situations
Bodily symptoms	The bodily sensations of panic (see below)
Associations	Strong association with panic disorder Secondary depression

- The condition may be severe and avoidance can lead the person to become housebound. Remarkably, symptoms (Table 10.4) are present for over 2 years on average before an agoraphobic seeks help. It is commonest in young women.
- For a vignette, see p. 68.

Social phobia
Social phobia (Table 10.5) must be distinguished from normal shyness, social withdrawal due to depression, or other psychiatric disorder. There is often a history of low self-esteem and a particular incident when the person feels they made a fool of themselves. Men and women are affected equally. Treatment is not well established; CBT or MAOIs are often used.

10.2.2 Panic disorder
Panic attacks are episodes of severe anxiety with prominent bodily symptoms (Table 10.6) (p. 27). In *panic disorder*, the attacks recur over a period of at least 1 month and are associated with fear of the attacks themselves.

The differential diagnosis of panic disorder is from panic attacks which only occur in specific feared situations (i.e. phobic anxiety) or which occur occasionally in other neuroses and depressive disorder. Also beware organic disorders producing paroxysmal anxiety such as phaeochromocytoma.
- CBT is effective. It is aimed at helping the patient see the symptoms as the result of anxiety and not as indicators of catastrophe. Antidepressant drugs are also effective, though patients often find them hard to tolerate.
- Aetiologically, there appears to be a lowered biological threshold for anxiety, and pre-existing cognitive distortions.
- See vignette, p. 53.

10.2.3 Generalized anxiety disorder
A syndrome of persistent anxiety that may fluctuate but is neither episodic (as with panic), situational (as with phobia) nor lifelong (as with a personality disorder) (Table 10.7).
- Treatment is based on the same pharmacological, psychological and stress-reducing methods as for other anxiety disorders — but there are relatively few trials of their efficacy.
- The genetic vulnerability to generalized anxiety disorder overlaps with that for depressive disorder.

Table 10.5 Symptoms of social phobia.

Component	Prominent features
Emotion	Situational anxiety in social gatherings
Cognition	Being judged negatively by others
Behaviour	Avoidance of social occasions
Bodily symptoms	Blushing, trembling
Associations	Secondary alcohol misuse Low self-esteem

Table 10.6 Symptoms of a panic attack.

Component	Prominent features
Emotion	Severe, incapacitating anxiety. Feeling depersonalized or derealized
Cognition	Of dying, going mad or otherwise losing control
Behaviour	Escape (e.g. rushing out of the room)
Bodily symptoms	Prominent symptoms and signs of sympathetic arousal (Table 10.2)
Associations	Depression, agoraphobia

Table 10.7 Symptoms of generalized anxiety disorder.

Component	Prominent features
Emotion	Anxiety
Cognition	Excessive, disproportionate unfocused worries
Behaviour	Easily startled, on edge
Bodily symptoms	Multiple chronic aches, tension
Associations	Depression

10.3 Obsessive–compulsive disorder (OCD)

Obsessions and compulsions were defined on p. 12. In OCD these symptoms are the most prominent and persistent feature (Table 10.8).

The differential diagnosis is from depressive disorder (in which obsessional symptoms are common), psychotic disorder (since obsessions can be hard to distinguish from delusions; p. 12) and anankastic personality disorder (p. 147).

• Drug therapy and behavioural treatments may be used individually or together. Tricyclic antidepressants and SSRIs are both effective; clomipramine is often chosen.

Table 10.8 Symptoms of obsessive–compulsive disorder (OCD).

Component	Prominent features
Emotion	Anxiety about the topic of the obsessional thought
Cognition	Preoccupation with obsession(s)
Behaviour	Compulsions
Bodily symptoms	Tension, especially if prevented from doing compulsive act
Associations	Depression
	Anankastic personality disorder (Chapter 15)
	Tourette's syndrome (Chapter 16.6.3)

• The prognosis untreated is poor. OCD patients are frequently used as cases in psychiatry exams.

• Aetiological factors include a genetic vulnerability, anankastic personality and social stressors. The condition is perpetuated by the avoidance of situations that trigger the obsessional concerns and the performance of rituals (the compulsions), both of which stop the anxiety habituating.

• OCD is equally common in men and women.

10.4 Reactions to stress

In the past, all neuroses were regarded as reactions to stress. Though this is no longer so, in some cases a stressor appears to be of such overwhelming importance that the disorder is classified as a 'reaction to stress'. The whole range of neurotic symptoms may occur, commonly a mixture of distress, anxiety, depression and somatic symptoms.

The types of stress reactions are:

• *acute stress reactions* — beginning and ending within hours or days of the stressor;

• *adjustment disorders* — beginning less acutely and lasting several months; and

• *post-traumatic stress disorder* (PTSD) — a delayed response to an extreme stress associated with particular symptoms.

10.4.1 Acute stress reactions

These are transient but severe emotional reactions immediately following an exceptional stressor (e.g. being raped). These states are colloquially referred to as 'nervous shock' (Table 10.9).

Differential diagnosis includes the initial stages of other neuroses, acute psychosis and organic disorders producing delirium. Management is by removal of the stressor (if possible), reassurance and support. A short course of benzodiazepines may be used.

• There is no evidence that 'debriefing' (talking to a therapist about the incident soon afterwards) prevents longer-term problems — some studies suggest it may even be harmful.

10.4.2 Adjustment disorders

These are more prolonged reactions to stress in which symptoms begin within a month of the stress and last no longer than 6 months (Table 10.10).

• Grief reactions (p. 93) and psychological reactions to physical illness are types of adjustment reaction.

Management includes removing continuing stressors, offering supportive psychotherapy (p. 71) and treating significant depressive or anxiety symptoms in the usual way.

10.4.3 Post-traumatic stress disorder (PTSD)

PTSD is a delayed response to an exceptionally severe event (e.g. serious road accident, major disaster). It became topical because of its prevalence in Vietnam war veterans, and more recently has been recognized as a basis for personal injury compensation claims. Onset is months or years after the trauma (Table 10.11).

Management includes treating any concurrent psychiatric disorder or substance misuse, and encouraging a return to normal activities. Antidepressants help reduce symptoms. There is some evidence for the effectiveness of CBT. A novel treatment called eye movement desensitization is of uncertain value. The prognosis is generally good with a gradual resolution in most cases.

10.5 Dissociative disorders

In dissociative disorders, also called *conversion disorders*, there is a medically inexplicable loss of function (Table 10.12). They are called dissociative because there is a loss of integration between personal identity and memories, sensory and motor function. Presentations include loss of memory (*psychogenic amnesia*),

Table 10.9 Symptoms of acute stress reaction.

Component	Prominent features
Emotion	'Dazed'
Cognition	Amnesia or denial of event
Behaviour	Overactivity, withdrawal
Somatic symptoms	Many autonomic symptoms

Table 10.10 Symptoms of adjustment disorders.

Component	Prominent features
Emotion	Depression, anxiety, poor concentration, irritability
Cognition	Preoccupation with event
Behaviour	Angry outbursts
Bodily symptoms	Moderate autonomic symptoms

Table 10.12 Symptoms of dissociative disorder.

Component	Prominent features
Emotion	May be suppressed, denial of anxiety
Cognition	Denial of impact of stressors
Behaviour	Loss of function
Bodily symptoms	Involving affected parts
Associations	Acute stressors, depression

Table 10.11 Symptoms of post-traumatic stress disorder (PTSD).

Component	Prominent features
Emotion	Anxiety and irritability; numb and detached
Cognition	Repeated reliving of the event in images ('flashbacks') and nightmares
Behaviour	Avoidance of situations associated with the trauma
Bodily symptoms	Exaggerated startle response
Associations	Substance misuse, depression

wandering in a trance (*fugue*), glove and stocking anaesthesia, paralysis and pseudoseizures (p. 134).
• The disorders are rare but cause difficulties in diagnosis and management.
• Dissociative disorders were previously known as *hysteria*; this archaic and sexist term (suggesting causation by a wandering uterus) has now been abandoned.

When the possibility of dissociative disorder is raised, consider the following:
• Physical causes for the loss of function must be excluded. This may require extensive investigation. Dissociative disorders (which originate in unconscious processes) must also be distinguished from *factitious disorder* in which symptoms are produced deliberately (p. 174). Deciding whether someone is feigning can, of course, be tricky. The other main differential diagnosis is of *somatoform disorder*.
• There should be a plausible 'psychogenic' explanation for the symptoms, in terms of internal conflicts or a traumatic life event. The term *conversion* reflects the theory that such feelings and anxieties get converted into symptoms, which are more tolerable, partly because the person benefits from them — so-called secondary gain.
• The person may be surprisingly unconcerned about their disability (*belle indifférence*).
• Management of acute cases involves acceptance of the reality of the patient's symptoms, together with encouragement toward recovery. Chronic cases may benefit from vigorous treatment of coexisting depression and from physical rehabilitation.

10.6 Somatoform disorders

In somatoform disorders (Table 10.13), the patient presents with medical complaints, either of symptoms for which there is no adequate medical explanation (*somatization*), or with the worry that they have a serious physical illness (*hypochondriasis*). To make the diagnosis the following conditions must be satisfied.

Table 10.13 Symptoms of somatoform disorders.

Component	Prominent features
Emotion	Anxiety and depression usually present (but not predominant)
Cognition	Concern with physical symptoms and/or disease
Behaviour	Medical help seeking
Bodily symptoms	Prominent
Associations	Depressive and anxiety disorders

• The concerns and/or symptoms are medically unjustified or disproportionate.
• The symptoms have persisted for at least 6 months.
• Anxiety and depressive symptoms are insufficient for a diagnosis of depressive or anxiety disorder.
• The symptoms are not delusional (cf. *delusional disorder*).
• The symptoms are not deliberately manufactured (cf. *factitious disorder*), nor is there loss of a specific function (cf. *dissociative disorder*).

Since patients (and perhaps their doctors) believe their symptoms are a sign of physical disease, they seek and receive medical rather than psychiatric care. Patients are often hostile to the idea that their symptoms are 'psychogenic' or that they will benefit from psychiatric treatment.
• The medical perspective on the relationship between somatic symptoms and psychiatric disorder is covered in Chapter 18.

Aetiologically, childhood deprivation or abuse appear to be risk factors. A predisposition to health anxiety and serious (and perhaps mismanaged) illness in a relative are also commonly observed.

Management of somatoform disorder requires close liaison between GP, physician and psychiatrist. The principles are:
• Take the patient's complaints seriously. Do not dismiss them, nor collude with inaccurate beliefs about their nature and origin.

• Investigations should be determined by the symptoms, not the patient's demands. People with somatoform disorder do not die of undiagnosed physical disease.

• Ensure a clear and consistent explanation for the symptoms is given by all doctors involved.

• Treat any coexisting depression and anxiety effectively.

• Identify and deal with major stressors.

• Encourage a return to normal functioning and decrease abnormal illness behaviour.

10.6.1 Hypochondriasis

The characteristic feature of this form of somatoform disorder is preoccupation with the possibility of having a serious physical disease. Patients repeatedly seek medical reassurance and investigation, but are not actually reassured by either.

• *Dysmorphophobia* is a form of hypochondriasis in which the preoccupation concerns physical appearance (e.g. perceived ugliness or deformity).

• The main differential diagnoses are depressive disorder (hypochondriacal worries are common) and psychotic disorders (with hypochondriacal delusions; p. 124).

• Management follows the principles described for somatoform disorder in general. CBT aimed at re-evaluating disease beliefs and fears is effective. The prognosis is variable: transient hypochondriasis is common (e.g. in medical students), but once established the condition can last many years and lead to extensive medical interventions.

10.6.2 Somatization disorders

Somatization refers to medically unexplained bodily symptoms, commonly pain, thought to have arisen from psychosocial stresses. We all somatize from time to time, but in *somatization disorder* the symptoms are persistent and dysfunctional.

• The terminology in this area is particularly muddled. Consult a larger text for details of specific somatization disorders.

• Somatization disorder is the psychiatric diagnosis for many patients with *functional* somatic syndromes such as irritable bowel syndrome and fibromyalgia. These patients comprise a third of all attenders at medical outpatient clinics, and are an important group (p. 173).

• Differential diagnosis is from the diseases that present with similar symptoms and from depressive and anxiety disorders. Also consider factitious disorder (p. 174).

• Management is based on the principles outlined for all somatoform disorders. Most patients respond to an extent to antidepressants. CBT is helpful for some of the specific somatization syndromes.

• Prognosis is very variable. Chronic disability is not uncommon.

Briquet's syndrome

Briquet's syndrome is severe, chronic somatization disorder. Patients, usually women, present with multiple medically unexplained symptoms over many years, and may have had all removable organs removed. They have been described as adopting illness as a way of life. Recurrent depression and personality disorder are common associations — indeed some regard Briquet's syndrome as a personality disorder.

• Management emphasizes containment rather than cure.

• Prognosis is very poor. Iatrogenic problems may result from the many medical interventions.

• In ICD-10, Briquet's syndrome is a synonym for somatization disorder as a whole. Our definition of it comes from DSM-IV and is more widely used in practice.

10.7 Neurasthenia

Neurasthenia is now often called *chronic fatigue syndrome*. It has much in common with somatoform disorders, in that physical complaints predominate and presentation is to non-psychiatric services. The main features are persistent, disabling fatigue and pain (Table 10.14).

Component	Prominent features
Emotion	Exhaustion, tiredness, irritability
Cognition	Concern about fatigue and its causes, poor concentration
Behaviour	Avoidance of physical exertion
Bodily symptom	Physical and/or mental fatigue after minor exertion Muscular pain (myalgia) Headache Patchy sleep
Associations	Depression

Table 10.14 Symptoms of neurasthenia.

• This constellation of symptoms has also been referred to as myalgic encephalomyelitis (ME). This term is misleading and best avoided.
• The main differential diagnosis is from medical disorders and depressive disorder.
• There is evidence for the efficacy of both CBT and antidepressants in neurasthenia.
• The prognosis is poor with a tendency towards chronicity. Avoidance of physical activity and excessive concern about the condition's causation are associated with a worse outcome.
• The aetiology is controversial. Both biological and psychological factors are involved. There is evidence for disturbed cerebral 5-HT function and social stress. Although many patients report onset after a viral infection, the aetiological role of viruses is uncertain.

10.8 Depersonalization-derealization syndrome

Depersonalization and derealization (p. 13) are neurotic symptoms. Occasionally they are the predominant feature, in which case this diagnostic category is used. The differential diagnosis is from a *depressive or anxiety disorder*, from *psychosis* and from *organic causes* especially *temporal lobe epilepsy* (p. 134). There is no specific therapy.

10.9 SUMMARY: KEY POINTS

• The neuroses are emotional disorders. Anxiety in one guise or another is the central feature.
• Neurotic symptoms also occur commonly in other psychiatric disorders.
• Neuroses afflict 15% of the population, women more than men. They may become chronic and disabling. The main subtypes are anxiety disorders and somatoform disorders.

• Somatoform disorders encompass medically unexplained symptoms (somatization) and fears about having physical disease (hypochondriasis). They are usually seen in non-psychiatric medical settings.
• Neuroses can be treated psychologically (with CBT) or with antidepressants. Anxiolytics are also effective and can be valuable in the short term.

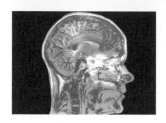

Eating, Sleep and Sexual Disorders

Disorders of eating, sleeping and sexuality are grouped together as syndromes associated with a disturbance in basic behaviours.

• Assessment of eating disorders was covered in a module (p. 29); assessment of sexual functioning is dealt with in this chapter.

11.1 Anorexia nervosa

11.1.1 Clinical features

The defining clinical features are:

• *Deliberate weight loss*, induced primarily by restriction of food intake.

• *Weight > 15% below normal* (BMI < 17.5; p. 29).

• A *dread of fatness* and *disturbance in perception of body weight* — the patient believes herself to be overweight when she isn't. The belief is an overvalued idea rather than a delusion (p. 12).

• *Amenorrhoea* (if not on the pill). Part of a wider endocrine disturbance which includes elevated cortisol and growth hormone levels.

Additional features include:

• A range of bodily symptoms and signs (Fig. 11.1).

• Depressive and obsessional symptoms.

• If the onset is before puberty, delay in secondary sexual development.

• A preoccupation with food and enjoyment of cooking for other people.

• Fatigue, irritability and coldness secondary to the weight loss.

• Social withdrawal and narrowing of interests.

• Use of diuretics, laxatives, excess exercise or self-induced vomiting to enhance weight loss.

Miss T, 14, was noticed to be losing weight although this was partially disguised by baggy clothing. She enjoyed cooking for the family and took up regular aerobics. She became vegetarian and avoided all fattening foods. When the issue of her weight was raised, Miss T became upset, insisting that she was fat. The GP found she was underweight (BMI = 14) and suspected anorexia nervosa.

Medical complications

The physical features of anorexia nervosa extend to serious medical complications, which are secondary to starvation and can be exacerbated by the effects of vomiting, diuretic and laxative abuse.

• Hypokalaemia is common and can cause fatal arrythmias.

• Hypotension, bradycardia, oedema, anaemia and cardiac failure.

• Hypoglycaemia.

• Osteoporosis.

• Hypothermia.

• Infections.

• Renal failure.

11.1.2 Epidemiology and aetiology

Anorexia mainly affects females (sex ratio 10 : 1). The average age of onset is 15–16 years. The prevalence in the UK is about 1% in females aged 12–18.

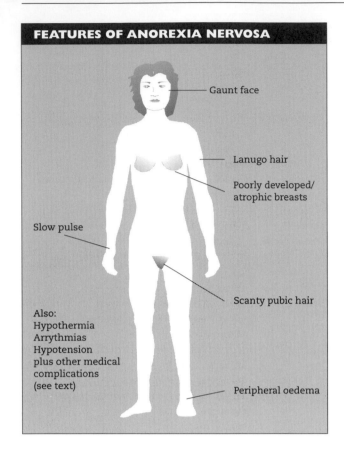

FEATURES OF ANOREXIA NERVOSA

Gaunt face

Lanugo hair

Poorly developed/
atrophic breasts

Slow pulse

Scanty pubic hair

Also:
Hypothermia
Arrythmias
Hypotension
plus other medical
complications
(see text)

Peripheral oedema

Fig. 11.1 Physical features of
anorexia nervosa.

Predisposing factors
• Moderate genetic contribution.
• Family history of depressive disorder, eating disorder or substance misuse.
• Personality traits of perfectionism, low self-esteem and excessive compliance.
• Families characterized by conflict avoidance, parental overinvolvement and a rigid structure.
• Anorexia is commoner in girls of higher social class, models and dancers.

Precipitating factors
• Critical comments about appearance—e.g. if premorbidly obese.
• Stressors during adolescence, such as school examinations and first sexual encounters.
• Dysfunction of central 5-HT receptors following normal dieting in vulnerable women.

Perpetuating factors
• The core psychological feature of anorexia nervosa—the fear of fatness—becomes paradoxically worse as weight is lost. Similarly, weight loss may enhance 5-HT dysfunction. The disorder is therefore self-perpetuating.
• Achieving a lower weight has certain rewards — it may enhance feelings of self-control, result in approval from peers, avoid sexual development or gain parental attention.

11.1.3 Differential diagnosis
The classic picture of anorexia nervosa is unmistakable. In the early stages it must be distinguished from other causes of weight loss. The psychiatric differential diagnoses include depressive disorder, substance misuse and obsessive–compulsive disorder; the

medical disorders include inflammatory bowel disease, malabsorption syndromes, hypopituitarism and cancer. The distinction is made by:
• detecting the core psychological symptoms of anorexia nervosa; and
• excluding physical and other psychiatric causes of weight loss.

11.1.4 Management

The management of anorexia nervosa involves:
• helping the patient increase weight;
• altering her attitude to weight and body shape via psychological treatments; and
• detecting and treating medical complications.

The first and third components can be achieved reasonably successfully, at least in the short term; the second component is more difficult as the core beliefs are often resistant to treatment.

Principles of management

• Establish a good therapeutic relationship — many patients are reluctant to accept treatment. Try to agree the goals:
    What weight is the person prepared to work towards?
    At what rate?
    How much exercise is appropriate?
• Encourage early weight gain to break the anorexic cycle and to overcome the problem that starvation interferes with psychological treatments. Weight gain is promoted by behavioural strategies — e.g. by contingent rewards.
• Low-dose antidepressants or antipsychotics are sometimes used to treat depressive or anxiety symptoms and to help weight gain.
• Psychotherapy involves education about the disorder and exploring issues which may have caused it or are perpetuating it. Psychodynamic methods are now being replaced by CBT. Both are of uncertain efficacy.
• Include the family in the educational and dietary aspects of care. Formal family therapy may be used, especially if the patient is still living in the parental home.

• Monitor physical condition. Serum potassium should be checked regularly.

Inpatient treatment

Inpatient care is indicated if anorexia nervosa is severe (e.g. weight < 65% of normal) or intractable. Consider compulsory admission if life is in immediate danger. Forced refeeding is used occasionally and controversially. Admission is preferably to a specialist unit. It usually lasts 8–12 weeks. The purposes of inpatient care are to:
• manage medical complications;
• actively encourage refeeding — ensuring a balanced diet of 3000 calories/day; and
• allow intensive psychological treatments.

Miss T is now 15 and has collapsed. For the past year, despite denials to her parents, she has eaten less than 1000 calories/day. She weighs 27 kg (BMI = 12), is hypothermic and has a low blood potassium. After medical stabilization she passively accepts admission to an eating disorder unit. She begins a behavioural programme with a target of gaining 0.5 kg/week for 2 months. A psychiatrist and nurse therapist explore eating and weight issues in individual and family sessions. Her potassium is monitored regularly. Ten weeks later her BMI is 15 and she becomes an outpatient.

11.1.5 Prognosis

Anorexia nervosa has a variable prognosis (Fig. 11.2).
• A long duration prior to presentation and an onset in adulthood predict poor outcome.
• Anorexia nervosa can develop into bulimia nervosa.
• There is a 20% mortality rate in long-term follow-up studies. Death is usually from complications of starvation, sometimes from suicide.

Miss T is now 27 and a beautician. She has a BMI of 15–16 and has occasional scanty menstrual periods. She continues to believe herself fat and gains self-esteem from her control over eating and weight. She restricts her intake to 1000 calories/day and works out daily. Now and then she

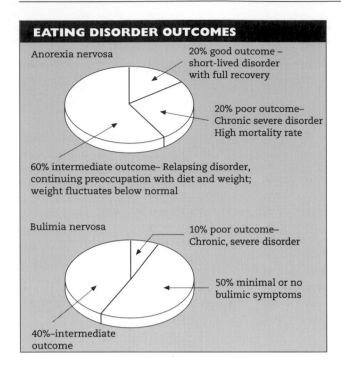

Fig. 11.2 Outcome in eating disorders.

has a large binge followed by self-induced vomiting and extra gym sessions. She avoids psychiatric care.

11.2 Bulimia nervosa

Bulimia refers to uncontrolled eating binges. Many people binge and feel bad about it, but in bulimia nervosa it is repetitive, excessive and associated with a preoccupation with weight control. Normal body weight is often maintained, at a price: self-induced vomiting and other means are used to negate the calorific effect of the binges.

11.2.1 Clinical features
Defining features
• Recurrent episodes of overeating (> twice a week) when large amounts are eaten in binges.
• Loss of control of eating during binges.
• Attempts to counteract the binges by vomiting, laxatives, enemas, diuretics, excessive exercise, etc.

• Preoccupation with body shape and weight.

Associated features
Vomiting and purging may lead to electrolyte disturbances, especially hypokalaemia, and a range of physical features:
• pitted teeth (eroded by gastric acid);
• calluses on knuckles (from putting fingers down throat);
• hoarse voice;
• parotid enlargement;
• seizures;
• tetany; and
• renal failure.

Miss V is a 23-year-old single woman. She has three or so episodes of overeating and vomiting a week. In an hour she can eat 10 packets of crisps, 10 chocolate bars and a couple of loaves of bread washed down with a bottle of wine. She then makes herself sick. She is preoccupied with her weight and shape and feels fat (though her BMI is normal). She first became concerned about her

*weight at the age of 14 when friends called her fat.
She was vegan for a while and is sometimes underweight and amenorrhoeic.*

11.2.2 Epidemiology and aetiology
Bulimia nervosa occurs in 2% of women aged
16–35 years but is otherwise rare. Only 10%
of cases ever present for help. Many of the
risk factors are shared with anorexia nervosa
(p. 106). The genetic predisposition overlaps
with that for panic disorder and phobic
anxiety. Other factors particularly associated
with bulimia nervosa include a history of
depressive disorder, conduct disorder, obesity,
early menarche and, probably, sexual abuse (p.
162).
• A small percentage of bulimia nervosa
occurs in women with personality disorder
who self-harm and misuse drugs or alcohol .

11.2.3 Differential diagnosis
Distinguish bulimia nervosa from:
• Milder bulimia-like problems — called *binge
eating disorder*. Compared to bulimia nervosa,
the latter is more common in men (a third of
cases) and affects a wider age range.
• Sporadic bingeing in other psychiatric disor-
ders (e.g. atypical depression; p. 87).
• Anorexia nervosa with bulimic features.
• Medical causes of bingeing or vomiting.

11.2.4 Management
Take a stepped approach to bulimia nervosa,
depending on the severity of the problem and
the patient's wishes. Admission is rarely
needed. Treatments are markedly more effective than in anorexia nervosa.
• Self-help manuals are a cost-effective and
increasingly used first-line treatment.
• CBT and interpersonal therapy (IPT; p. 70)
are effective in 60–70% of patients, with the
majority remaining well 5 years later. CBT aims
to help the patient:
  — (a) understand the links between bingeing, vomiting and dieting;
  — (b) regulate their diet and break the
vicious cycle between the three behaviours;
and

  — (c) decrease their preoccupation with
body shape. IPT emphasizes the role of
relationship problems in the disorder.
• Fluoxetine reduces the frequency of bingeing
and vomiting. A high dose (60–80 mg/day) may
be required and the disorder often relapses on
stopping.

11.2.5 Prognosis
The prognosis of bulimia nervosa is uncertain
but probably better than that of anorexia
nervosa (Fig. 11.2). Poor prognostic factors
include coincidental personality disorder and
a long duration of bulimia prior to treatment.

11.3 Sleep disorders

Sleep problems are usually secondary to a psychiatric or medical disorder, but sometimes a
sleep disorder is the primary diagnosis.

11.3.1 Insomnia
Assessment
Insomnia describes a persistently unsatisfactory quantity or quality of sleep. A quarter of
adults complain of it. It causes much distress
and is a risk factor for premature death.
• Eighty per cent of cases of insomnia are
related to anxiety and depressive disorders.
Most of the rest are secondary to medical
disease, chronic pain and substance misuse.
The remaining fraction (< 10%) are *primary
insomnia*. To distinguish these cases, exclude
the presence of an underlying psychiatric or
medical disorder. Ask about other factors
which affect sleep such as shift working,
medication, alcohol, caffeine, etc. A sleep diary
and corroboration from the sleeping partner
are helpful.

Treatment
Treat any associated disorder (e.g. use a
sedative antidepressant if insomnia is due
to depression). Interventions for insomnia
include:
• *Stimulus control*. An effective method to
restore a good sleep routine. The person

should go to bed only when sleepy, put the light out straight away, get up if awake for more than 20 minutes, get up at a regular time and avoid daytime naps.
• *Sleep hygiene*. This approach pays attention to health practices (e.g. use of caffeine and alcohol) and stimuli (e.g. noise, light) which affect sleep.
• *Relaxation therapy*. Behavioural, cognitive and biofeedback routines to reduce arousal. The person should wind down 90 minutes before bedtime and practise relaxation when in bed.
• *Hypnotics*. Effective in the short term and widely used.

11.3.2 Hypersomnia

Hypersomnia is excessive daytime sleepiness, or having a prolonged time in the twilight zone between sleep and wakefulness. The term excludes cases secondary to insomnia or where there are clear reasons for such behaviour (e.g. shift working). Causes are shown in Table 11.1.
• In *narcolepsy* there are repeated attacks of daytime somnolence usually leading irresistibly to sleep. It is associated with *cataplexy* (abrupt loss of muscle tone), *hypnagogic hallucinations* (p. 13) and *sleep paralysis* (the patient wakes but is unable to move). Ninety-eight per cent have the DR15 variant of HLA-DR2. Stimulants are used for the somnolence and clomipramine for the cataplexy.

Table 11.1 Causes of hypersomnia.

Psychiatric disorders Depressive disorder Neurasthenia
Medical disorders Narcolepsy Kleine–Levin syndrome Sleep apnoea syndrome Chronic physical disease
Other Side-effects of drugs (prescribed or illicit)

11.3.3 Parasomnias

Parasomnias are abnormal episodic events during sleep — sleepwalking, nightmares, etc. They are part of normal development in children; in adults they usually reflect emotional stress.
• Distinguish parasomnias from other causes of odd nocturnal behaviour, such as epilepsy.

11.4 Sexual problems

An understanding of sexual problems and how to assess them is important in psychiatry because:
• Sexual dysfunction is a common consequence of psychiatric disorders or their treatment — for example, loss of libido in depression; ejaculatory failure due to antipsychotics.
• Sexual dysfunction may contribute to psychiatric disorder. For example, an anxiety disorder may be exacerbated by a man worrying about his impotence.
• Psychiatrists treat sexual dysfunction.
• Disorders of gender identity and sexual preference are psychiatric disorders.

11.4.1 Sexual dysfunction

Each of the components of sex — desire, physiological arousal, orgasm — can go awry (Table 11.2). Each type of dysfunction may be due to psychological or medical causes or both.
• Sexual desire and orgasmic disorders are commoner in women; the main problems for men are impotence and premature ejaculation.
• Sexual dysfunction is associated with sexual inexperience, anxiety and relationship problems.

Assessment of sexual dysfunction

Asking about sex is the topic that most health professionals feel least confident and most embarrassed about. This is unnecessary. Many patients are glad to be asked, since sexual problems are common and it may be their

Table 11.2 Types of sexual dysfunction.

Sexual desire disorders
Lack of
Excess

Failure of genital response
Erectile dysfunction (impotence)
Vaginal dryness

Orgasmic dysfunction
Premature ejaculation
Anorgasmia

Other
Vaginismus (involuntary spasm of vaginal
    musculature)
Dyspareunia (pain on intercourse)

first opportunity to seek reassurance or treatment.
• Know when to introduce the subject — try and respond to cues. For example, if a depressed patient tells you he gets no pleasure from life, it is a good moment to ask whether this has also affected his interest in sex. If no cue presents itself, preface the assessment with a comment such as: 'I need to ask you some questions about your sex life, to help me understand X. . . . Is this all right?'.
• Use terminology appropriate to the person's age and culture. For example, 'coming' and 'gay' are suitable for a teenager, but 'ejaculating' and 'homosexual' would be better for an elderly vicar.
    Assessment of sexual function covers several areas (Table 11.3). Some of the questions will be used regularly, others rarely.

Psychological treatment of sexual dysfunction
Sexual problems may respond to reassurance or use of self-help manuals. Others require sex therapy, which is provided by some psychiatrists and by private therapists. Sex therapy uses behavioural methods, and is effective (assuming no underlying medical cause for the dysfunction). The principles are as follows:
• Treat the couple together.

• Educate about sex and the factors affecting it.
• Encourage open discussion of feelings and decrease anxiety and embarrassment.
• Use graded exposure (p. 67). The couple gradually rebuild their sexual relationship, setting aside time and committing themselves to follow a series of steps — starting with non-genital 'sensate focus', then moving on via genital focus before finally returning to full intercourse. Additional methods are used for specific forms of dysfunction. For example, dilators for vaginismus, the squeeze technique for premature ejaculation.

11.4.2 Other sexual disorders
In these disorders the problem is not sex itself but the object of sexual desire—at least to the extent that it conflicts with society or causes harm. The person may or may not agree with this view. In ICD-10, these disorders are grouped with personality disorders.
• Forensic psychiatrists may be asked to report on the psychiatric status of sex offenders.
• Homosexuality is no longer classified as a psychiatric disorder.

Gender identity disorders
• In *transsexualism* the person, usually male, wishes to live as a member of the opposite sex. They seek hormonal or surgical treatment to match their body to their subjective gender. Sexual orientation is variable and sexual desire often low. Transsexuals may despair of their plight and depression is common.
• *Transvestism* is the urge to dress in clothes of the opposite sex. If accompanied by sexual arousal it is called *fetishistic transvestism*. There is no desire to change sex. Transvestites are often married and cross-dress secretly. There is no specific treatment.

Disorders of sexual preference (paraphilias)
Sexual desire can centre on a wide range of animate and inanimate objects. Such pleasures only constitute a disorder if the activity is illegal (e.g. paedophilia) or if sex becomes dys-

Table 11.3 Assessment of sexual function.

Questions	Comments
CURRENT SEXUAL FUNCTIONING	
What is the nature and frequency of sex?	
Is there a particular problem?	Get a history of each difficulty
How much interest do you have in sex?	Increased libido is rarely complained of.
Has this changed recently?	Occurs in mania
In men	
Erectile function:	
Any problems getting or keeping an erection?	
Do you get erections in the morning?	Loss of morning erections or of erection when masturbating suggests medical cause
Do you worry about your sexual performance?	Impotence often associated with performance anxiety
Ejaculatory function:	
Do you come too quickly?	Common in inexperienced, anxious men
How long after penetration?	
Do you feel anxious about this?	
In women	
Do you have pain on intercourse. Where? When?	Dyspareunia and vaginal dryness have psychological and gynaecological causes
Do you feel anxious or tense about sex?	Extreme anxiety can lead to vaginismus
SEXUAL DEVELOPMENT	
Estimate age of puberty	Problems or delays in sexual development may lead to psychological effects or indicate an
When did your voice break?	
Periods start?	abnormality (e.g. Turner's syndrome)
When did you first masturbate? First have intercourse?	Affected by cultural and individual differences
SEXUAL ORIENTATION AND PREFERENCES	
What is their sexual orientation?	This should have been recorded in the core assessment
Does he have particular sexual preferences or fetishes?	Detailed questioning indicated if the patient views it as a problem, or in a forensic context
If so, what?	
Have they ever got you into trouble?	
OTHER ISSUES	
Current psychiatric disorder?	Psychiatric disorders, especially depression, associated with sexual dysfunction
General health?	Medical disorders (e.g. diabetes, vascular disease) affect sexual functioning. Do physical examination
Current medication?	Many drugs have sexual side-effects

functional and overdependent on an object (e.g. fetishism). Paraphilia is almost exclusively a male disorder.

• In *paedophilia*, sexual interest or activity centres on prepubescent children. The prevalence is unknown, though there is a considerable demand for child pornography. Psychological treatments have been used to reduce reoffending rates; cyproterone acetate, an antiandrogen, has been used to suppress libido. The effectiveness of these treatments is uncertain.

• *Exhibitionism* is the exposing of the genitals to strangers. Two groups are recognized: inhibited men who struggle against the urge, feel guilty and expose a flaccid penis (type 1); and aggressive men who expose an erect penis and masturbate then or later (type 2). The latter shows an association with actual sexual assaults. Behavioural treatments may be beneficial.

11.5 SUMMARY: KEY POINTS

• In anorexia nervosa there is weight loss, fear of fatness and amenorrhoea. In bulimia nervosa there are episodes of uncontrollable binge eating and vomiting, and a preoccupation with weight and food. Both occur mainly in young women. Bulimia nervosa responds well to psychological treatments, anorexia nervosa less so.

• Sleep disorders comprise insomnia (not enough), hypersomnia (too much) and parasomnias (disturbances during sleep). They may be treated psychologically or pharmacologically.

• Sexual dysfunction is common and can affect desire, the mechanics of arousal, or orgasm. Assessment of sexual function is important. Sex therapy is effective for many of the problems.

CHAPTER 12

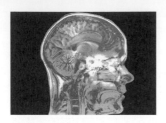

Schizophrenia

12.1 Clinical features of schizophrenia

Schizophrenia is the disorder at the heart of specialist psychiatry and is closest to the public conception of madness. It is distinguished from other psychoses by:
• the presence of specific types of delusion, hallucination and thought disorder;
• the clinical course; and
• the absence of a mood disorder or organic psychosis.

The clinical picture of schizophrenia is complex and heterogeneous. In this section, the features characterizing the acute and the chronic stages of the disorder are described in turn.

12.1.1 Clinical features of acute schizophrenia

Of the features in Table 12.1, particular weight is placed on the presence of the first-rank symptoms (p. 22). However, diagnosis does not depend on a certain number of the features being present; rather, the more there are, the more likely schizophrenia becomes.
• Before proceeding, review the psychosis module (p. 19) and relevant parts of the core assessment (p. 9). These earlier sections include definitions of the cardinal symptoms.

• The duration criterion is to exclude transient schizophrenia-like syndromes which have a better prognosis (and maybe a different aetiology). If the features of schizophrenia are present but for less than a month, the label is *schizophreniform disorder*.
• Schizophrenia beginning after the age of 45 used to be considered a separate disorder, *paraphrenia*.

Clinical subtypes of schizophrenia
For descriptive purposes, schizophrenia is divided into four subsyndromes (Table 12.2).
• The catatonic subtype is rarer than it used to be. This could reflect a change in the nature or treatment of the disease, or the past occurrence of neurological disorders mistaken for schizophrenia (particularly a postviral condition called encephalitis lethargica).

Mr J is a 20-year-old student found having a conversation with imaginary demons. His room was covered in black paper to stop them interfering with his thoughts. His work had deteriorated markedly in the past term, and he had isolated himself. He was convinced that he was part of a sinister plot and was being told what to do by unknown people whom he could hear talking about him. There was no evidence of substance misuse or mood disorder. A provisional diagnosis of paranoid schizophrenia was made.

12.1.2 Clinical features of chronic schizophrenia

In patients who progress to chronic schizophrenia, the predominant picture is of a 'burnt-out' disease (Table 12.3). These features are called *negative symptoms*, in contrast to the *positive symptoms* of Table 12.1.

Table 12.1 Clinical features of acute schizophrenia.

> *Characteristic symptoms*
> First-rank symptoms
>   Thought insertion, echo, withdrawal or
>   broadcasting
>   Third person auditory hallucinations
>   'Running commentary' hallucinations
>   Passivity of thought, feelings or action
>   Delusional perception
> Bizarre delusions
> Odd behaviour
> Thought disorder
> Lack of insight (reality distortion)
> Prodromal period of decline in performance
>   and social withdrawal
>
> *Duration criterion*
> Symptoms present for at least 1 month
>
> *Major exclusion criteria*
> Not secondary to elevation or depression of
>   mood
> No demonstrable organic cause (e.g.
>   amphetamine abuse, temporal lobe
>   epilepsy)

• Prominent, enduring negative symptoms are labelled *deficit syndrome*.

• The positive–acute, negative–chronic distinction is not absolute — positive symptoms regularly occur in chronic cases, and some patients have negative symptoms in their first episode.

• *Residual schizophrenia* is a transitional state between acute and chronic schizophrenia. It describes patients with positive symptoms within the past year who have also developed negative symptoms.

Mr J is now 45. He has had multiple admissions. Between episodes, he never regained his previous level of functioning; by 35 he was living in a group home (p. 119). He spends most of his time in his room or walking the streets, often mumbling to himself. He has no specific

Table 12.3 Features of chronic schizophrenia.

> *Negative symptoms*
> Flattened (blunted) mood
> Apathy and loss of drive (avolition)
> Social isolation
> Poverty of speech
> Poor self-care
>
> *Other features*
> Positive symptoms persist or recur at times of
>   stress
> Mild cognitive impairment is common

Table 12.2 Subtypes of acute schizophrenia.

Subtype	Predominant symptoms	Other features
Paranoid	Persecutory, systematized delusions Hallucinations, usually auditory	Commonest form Personality relatively preserved
Disorganized (hebephrenic)	Thought disorder Odd behaviour Fleeting, bizarre delusions Labile or inappropriate mood	Early onset Poor prognosis Premorbid personality often schizoid or schizotypal
Catatonic	Motor signs (see p. 20)	Now rare in developed countries
Undifferentiated	A mixture of the above	

complaints or desires. His last admission was a year ago when hallucinations recurred following another resident's suicide.

• Recently the symptoms of chronic schizophrenia have been shown to fall more clearly into three clusters, rather than the two implied by the positive–negative distinction. The three are *reality distortion* (delusions and hallucinations), *disorganization* (thought disorder) and *psychomotor poverty* (similar to negative symptoms).

12.2 Differential diagnosis of schizophrenia

12.2.1 Acute schizophrenia

Acute schizophrenia must be distinguished from other psychotic disorders (Table 12.4).
• Drug-induced psychoses pose a particular problem. More than 30% of people with schizophrenia misuse alcohol or drugs, and it can be difficult to decide whether these constitute the 'cause' of their symptoms. Judgement is based on the timing, quantity and type of substances taken.

• The organic disorders which can produce an acute schizophrenic picture (sometimes called *symptomatic schizophrenia*) are collectively common enough — about 5% of cases — to require a high index of suspicion, especially if aspects of the case are atypical.

12.2.2 Chronic schizophrenia

In chronic schizophrenia the diagnosis itself is rarely in doubt, though occasionally neurological syndromes (e.g. a leukodystrophy) can mimic the clinical picture.
• A commoner problem is the need to distinguish negative symptoms from depression or from the sedative and parkinsonian effects of antipsychotics (p. 63).

12.2.3 Investigations in schizophrenia

Schizophrenia is a clinical diagnosis. Physical investigations are mainly used to rule out the organic disorders in Table 12.4, and are chosen according to the features elicited in the history and examination.
• Brain imaging is not routine. It should be considered if there are neurological symptoms or signs.

Table 12.4 Differential diagnosis of acute schizophrenia.

Category of disorder	Distinguishing features/examples
Other non-organic disorders	
Delusional disorders	Absence of specific features of schizophrenia
Psychotic depression	Prominent depressive symptoms
Manic episode	Prominent manic symptoms
Schizoaffective disorder	Mood and schizophrenia symptoms both prominent
Schizotypal disorder	Nature of symptoms; chronic history
Puerperal psychosis	Acute onset after childbirth
Organic disorders	
Drug-induced psychosis	History of drug or alcohol misuse
Side-effects of therapeutic drugs	L-dopa, methyldopa, steroids, antimalarials
Temporal lobe epilepsy	Other evidence of seizures
Delirium	Acute onset, clouding of consciousness
Dementia	Age, known cognitive impairment
Head injury	History
Huntington's disease	Family history; choreiform movements, dementia
HIV	Positive HIV test
Systemic lupus erythematosus	Skin and renal involvement
Syphilis	Other evidence of infection

12.3 Epidemiology of schizophrenia

The lifetime risk for schizophrenia is about 0.8%, with an annual incidence of 1–2 per 10 000 and a point prevalence of 50 per 10 000.
• Onset peaks in early adulthood, and is somewhat later in women than men (Fig. 12.1).
• There is an equal sex ratio, but men tend to have a worse prognosis.

Two findings about the recent incidence of schizophrenia in the UK are notable:
• The incidence has fallen over the past 30 years. It is unclear how much of this is an artefact of changes in diagnostic criteria or admission rates.
• There is an increased frequency (relative risk ~5) of schizophrenia in the children of Afro-Caribbeans who migrated to Britain in the 1950s. Its explanation is controversial, with biological (genetic, viral) and sociological (racial prejudice, social deprivation) theories.

12.4 Management of schizophrenia

The management of schizophrenia can be considered according to the stage of the illness (acute vs. chronic) or to the intervention (physical, psychological, social).

12.4.1 Management of acute schizophrenia

The key elements are summarized in Table 12.5.

Admission is usual. The Mental Health Act may be needed, since patients are at risk from neglect or dangerous acts. Ideally, there should be several days of drug-free observation; this is rarely feasible due to shortage of beds or because the behaviour is too disturbed. Antipsychotics are effective against positive symptoms in a majority (~75%) of patients over 2–3 weeks. During this period, add benzodiazepines if behaviour is difficult to manage or the patient is very distressed (p. 62).
• Investigate the context of the disorder (pp. 13, 22), as it may give clues as to its development and prognosis.
• Involve the family. Relatives need support and explanation; they may also be a therapeutic target (p. 119).
• First admissions can last many weeks depending on progress and external factors (e.g. finding accommodation). Future management is planned at predischarge care programme approach (CPA) meetings (p. 80).

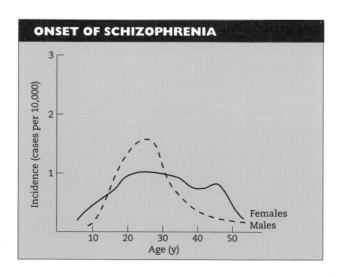

Fig. 12.1 Schizophrenia: age at onset.

Table 12.5 Components in the management of acute schizophrenia.

Intervention	Rationale
Admission	For diagnosis, investigation, and starting treatment
Antipsychotic drugs	For treatment of symptoms
Benzodiazepines	For sedation
Establish context of disorder	
Evaluate current personal circumstances	To guide management—accommodation, work, etc.
Assessment of needs and of risk	
Education of patient and family	To improve understanding and treatment adherence

• Following a schizophrenic episode, *post-schizophrenic depression* is common.

12.4.2 Management of chronic schizophrenia

After a first episode of schizophrenia, the aims are:
• to prevent relapse; and
• to optimize level of functioning.
To do this, a combination of pharmacological, psychological and social methods is used (Table 12.6). The amount of intervention needed varies markedly, depending on the course and severity of the disorder. In this section, the emphasis is on cases where full recovery has not occurred after the first episode.

The most important specific intervention is antipsychotic medication, which reduces the rate of relapse in the 2 years after an episode from 70% to 50%. Even the benefits of psychological and family interventions may operate partly by improving treatment adherence. Equally, however, a sustained relationship must be established with the patient and due atten-

tion paid to their 'problems of living'. Without this commitment, the patient is unlikely to comply with any management plan.
• The value of a multidisciplinary approach is apparent from the range of patients' needs — benefits, accommodation, employment, physical health, etc. The nature of the disorder, especially the effect of negative symptoms, makes people with chronic schizophrenia vulnerable in all these areas.

12.4.3 Modes of treatment for schizophrenia

Antipsychotic drugs

After a single episode of schizophrenia, continue medication for 12–24 months. If the person remains well it should then be tailed off because there is little evidence that further medication is beneficial and because of the risk of tardive dyskinesia (p. 63). Patients who have had multiple episodes or persistent symptoms usually remain on medication for many years, though the need for it (and the effect of cautious reductions in dose) should remain

Table 12.6 Components in the management of chronic schizophrenia.

Intervention	Rationale
Care programme approach	To ensure medical and social needs are met
Maintenance of antipsychotic medication	To prevent relapse
Readmission during severe relapses	To stabilize mental state and review management
Family therapy for high expressed emotion	To prevent relapse
Social skills training	To improve social functioning
Cognitive therapy	To reduce symptoms, increase treatment adherence

under regular review. Medication is often given in depot form (p. 64).

• A third of patients are resistant to, or intolerant of, typical antipsychotics. Clozapine and other atypical antipsychotics are alternatives; they have benefits, but their role is not yet clear (p. 65).

• Persistent negative symptoms (Table 12.3) are not improved by antipsychotics. Conversely, neither do the drugs cause them.

Other physical treatments

• Benzodiazepines are useful for short-term sedation.

• Antidepressants should be used if depression occurs in schizophrenia.

• Electroconvulsive therapy (ECT) is rarely used, except for catatonic stupor and as a last resort in drug-resistant cases.

Psychological treatments

The main specific psychological intervention is a form of family therapy. This arose from the finding that patients living with families who have *high expressed emotion* (EE) had a much higher chance of relapse than those exposed to low EE. EE is the intensity and amount of emotional involvement by the family with the patient. It was then found that high EE families could be taught to lower EE, and relapse rates fell. Such family intervention is only moderately effective; several families have to be treated to prevent one relapse.

• The converse of high EE — a lack of stimulation — is also harmful as it exacerbates the apathy and withdrawal of chronic schizophrenia. This was first documented in institutionalized patients (and contributed to the drive to close the asylums).

• Supportive psychotherapy (p. 71) of patients and their families should be part of the care package.

• Cognitive therapy is effective for some symptoms such as drug-resistant delusions. These can also benefit from simple manoeuvres such as ear plugs and personal stereos.

Social interventions

The nature of chronic schizophrenia means that many patients have problems with daily living. These needs should be identified and met by the community mental health team (CMHT; p. 76). The reality is, however, that some patients slip through the net, with largely invisible but occasionally tragic consequences.

• Some patients cannot live alone or with their family. *Group homes* are houses where several patients live together, supported by their key worker and the group homes organization.

Ms C is a 28-year-old factory worker who's had one episode of schizophrenia. She was discharged home under the care of her CMHT on a depot. A CPN visited to monitor progress, give medication and advise the parents about how best to interact with Ms C. After discussion with her employers, Ms C returned to work part-time but 3 months later she refused medication and began smoking cannabis. She relapsed and lost her job, and her behaviour became unmanageable. She was readmitted. Once her condition had settled, a meeting was held between Ms C, her parents and the CMHT. Ms C was offered a place in a group home. She agreed to take medication regularly. She was found sheltered employment in a charity shop. The CMHT social worker helped sort out Ms C's financial problems and ensured that she got her benefits.

12.5 Prognosis of schizophrenia

Accurate estimates for the long-term outcome of schizophrenia are surprisingly hard to obtain, because the diagnostic criteria have changed over time and because they depend on how recovery is defined. For example, some patients have persistent symptoms but live a reasonably normal life; others are functionally impaired despite minimal symptoms. Taking both symptoms and functioning into account, only about a third of cases have the stereotype of a chronic, deteriorating course;

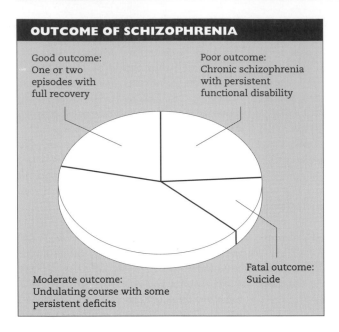

OUTCOME OF SCHIZOPHRENIA

Good outcome:
One or two
episodes with
full recovery

Poor outcome:
Chronic schizophrenia
with persistent
functional disability

Moderate outcome:
Undulating course with some
persistent deficits

Fatal outcome:
Suicide

Fig. 12.2 Outcomes of schizophrenia.

Table 12.7 Factors associated with a poor outcome in schizophrenia.

Demographic characteristics
Young age at onset (e.g. under 25)
Male
Isolated, unmarried
Poor work record
Premorbid personality disorder
Substance misuse

Illness characteristics
Insidious onset
Prolonged untreated psychosis
Disorganized subtype
No mood disturbance
Negative symptoms

a quarter have a very good outcome, and the remaining half have a relapsing, remitting illness (Fig. 12.2).
• About 10% commit suicide. The risk is higher after an acute episode, when the patient may have realized the nature of his disorder and its implications, and may have developed a depressive disorder.

Poor outcome factors are shown in Table 12.7. However, they are only weak predictors and it is impossible to foresee which category

in Fig. 12.2 someone presenting with schizophrenia will end up in.
• First-rank symptoms have no prognostic significance.
• The outcome of schizophrenia appears to be better in developing than developed countries, presumably reflecting the importance of the social environment.

12.6 Aetiology of schizophrenia

There have been many and diverse views of schizophrenia: as a brain disease; as a psychological disorder with no organic basis; and as a myth. Over the past 20 years, its original conception as a genetically driven neurodevelopmental disorder again prevails.

12.6.1 Genetic factors

There is an increased risk of schizophrenia in people with a family history of the disease (Fig. 12.3). Adoption and twin studies (p. 55) show that this is due to genetic factors. The mode of inheritance is not clear. It probably involves several genes interacting with each other (one

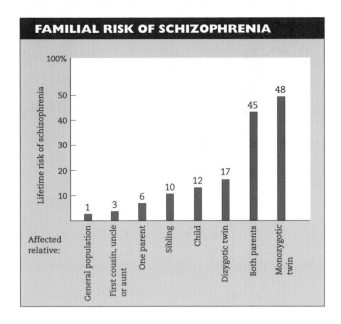

Fig. 12.3 Familial risks of schizophrenia.

may be on chromosome 6) and with the environmental influences mentioned below.

• Family studies show that the schizophrenia genes overlap with those for schizotypal disorder and delusional disorder (p. 123). These conditions are therefore sometimes grouped together as *schizophrenia spectrum disorders*.

12.6.2 Environmental factors

Genes are not the sole cause of schizophrenia — 70% of cases do not have an affected relative and the concordance amongst identical twins is < 50%. The putative environmental risk factors are obstetric — e.g. maternal influenza and birth complications. They are of minor effect compared to the genetic contribution, but cumulatively support the view that schizophrenia has its roots in early development.

12.6.3 The brain in schizophrenia
Neurochemical findings

The pre-eminent *dopamine hypothesis* proposes that schizophrenia is due to excess dopaminergic function in the limbic system. It is supported by the findings that:

• antipsychotic drugs are potent dopamine receptor antagonists;
• dopamine agonists (e.g. amphetamines) produce a paranoid psychosis; and
• some post-mortem studies in schizophrenia have found increased dopamine D_2 and D_4 receptors.

However, though dopaminergic abnormalities may well contribute to the clinical features, a causal role now seems unlikely because:

• the D_2 receptor increase is largely a result of antipsychotics given to patients;
• imaging of D_2 receptors in first-episode patients has not shown consistent abnormalities;
• the dopamine receptor genes are not associated with schizophrenia; and
• amphetamine psychosis is not really like schizophrenia.

Attention has now turned to other neurotransmitter systems. In particular, the effects of phencyclidine (PCP; p. 144) suggest glutamatergic hypofunction in schizophrenia.

Functional imaging studies

Localized abnormalities in cerebral blood flow

and glucose metabolism occur in schizophrenia. For example, patients:
• fail to activate the prefrontal cortex when performing tasks requiring its use (*hypofrontality*);
• show abnormal blood-flow responses to dopaminergic drugs; and
• have characteristic metabolic patterns depending on their predominant symptoms.

Neuropathological findings

The most robust finding, confirmed by meta-analysis, is enlargement of the lateral ventricles and a corresponding decrease in cortical volume. There may be a preferential involvement of the temporal lobe and a loss of normal cerebral asymmetries.

Fig. 12.4 The neurodevelopmental model of schizophrenia.

• The histological basis of schizophrenia is unknown, though the cytoarchitecture of the cerebral cortex — its neuronal organization — appears altered. There is no gliosis (see below).

12.6.4 Psychological and social theories

The earlier psychological and social (p. 52) theories of the causation of schizophrenia lack supporting evidence. However, such factors are clearly important in its outcome, exemplified by the effect of EE (p. 119); they may also be relevant in the onset of schizophrenia, since there is an excess of life events in the months preceding the first episode.
• Psychological interest is now directed mainly at the neuropsychological mechanisms. For example, one theory views schizophrenia as affecting the ability to distinguish actions generated by internal events (thoughts, feelings) and external stimuli (sensations).

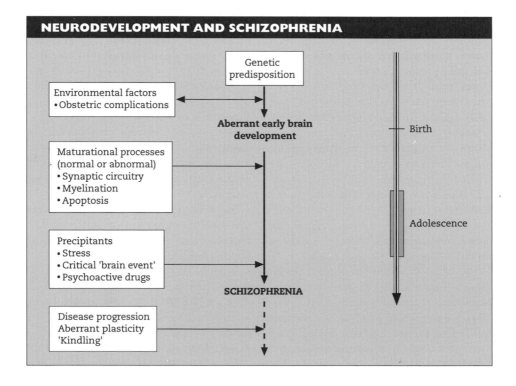

NEURODEVELOPMENT AND SCHIZOPHRENIA

Genetic predisposition

Environmental factors
• Obstetric complications

Aberrant early brain development

Birth

Maturational processes (normal or abnormal)
• Synaptic circuitry
• Myelination
• Apoptosis

Adolescence

Precipitants
• Stress
• Critical 'brain event'
• Psychoactive drugs

SCHIZOPHRENIA

Disease progression Aberrant plasticity 'Kindling'

12.6.5 The neurodevelopmental model

Schizophrenia appears to be the result of an anomaly of brain development, driven by a genetic predisposition and early environmental factors (Fig. 12.4). As evidence in favour of the neurodevelopmental model:

• The ventricular enlargement is present at the onset of symptoms and is largely static thereafter.

• The lack of gliosis and cytoarchitectural abnormalities suggest a prenatal origin.

• The environmental risk factors act *in utero*.

• Children destined as adults to get schizophrenia have impaired behavioural, intellectual and motor development, demonstrable from infancy onwards.

Though psychological and social factors do not play major roles in the model, their influence should not be ignored, as mentioned above. These are likely to be mediated via stress and its effects upon neural plasticity.

12.7 Disorders related to schizophrenia

Several other disorders are grouped together with schizophrenia, because:

• they are all psychoses which are not secondary to a mood disorder or organic disorder (in the case of schizoaffective disorder and delusional disorders); or

• they are thought to be causally related (in the case of schizotypal disorder).

12.7.1 Schizoaffective disorder

Clinical features

The distinction of schizophrenia from bipolar disorder originated in the belief that these were two discrete disorders, and is reflected in the classification of bipolar disorder as a mood disorder separate from schizophrenia (p. 4). However, this view is probably wrong. Certainly many patients have features of both conditions, hence *schizoaffective disorder*.

• Limit the diagnosis to individuals who satisfy criteria for schizophrenia *and* mood disorder

occurring during the same episode. Otherwise, diagnose the predominant syndrome. For example, one first-rank symptom in mania does not warrant a label of schizoaffective disorder (let alone schizophrenia). Similarly, labile mood is common in acute schizophrenia.

Management and prognosis

Mood symptoms and schizophrenic symptoms are treated on their merits. Lithium and antipsychotics are often used in combination.

• The prognosis is intermediate between schizophrenia and mood disorder. It is better in those whose predominant mood disturbance is manic rather than depressive. Deficit syndrome (p. 115) is rarely seen.

12.7.2 Delusional disorders (paranoid psychoses)

Many patients have a psychosis without an underlying mood disturbance or organic disorder but do not satisfy the criteria for schizophrenia. Persecutory (paranoid) delusions are the main feature. Hallucinations are rare and personality remains intact.

• The disorders in this 'residual' category of psychosis have had a variety of names. The preferred collective term is now *delusional disorder*, though *paranoid psychosis* is still commonly used.

Acute delusional disorder

These conditions are characterized by their acute onset, clinical features and rapid resolution. There are multiple, transient persecutory delusions, and there is a sense of perplexity or suspicion and a labile mood.

• They may be caused by drugs (in which case they are diagnosed as such) or follow extreme stresses, hence the older terms *psychogenic psychosis* and *brief reactive psychosis*.

Persistent delusional disorder

A *persistent delusional disorder* is one lasting more than 3 months. *Chronic paranoid psychosis* and *paranoia* describe similar disorders.

• The delusions are *systematized* (i.e. stable and combined into a complex system). They often centre upon alleged (and plausible) injustices. The person may embark on litigation, or occasionally retribution, so it is important to ask about thoughts of aggression and hostility.

• The delusions are often *encapsulated*. The rest of the mental state can be unremarkable to the point that, if the delusional system is not detected, no abnormal features are elicited. Because of this, the disorder can go unrecognized for years, becoming hard to distinguish from paranoid personality disorder (p. 147) — though in the latter the paranoid ideas are not truly delusional.

• Social isolation, deafness and paranoid personality traits are risk factors.

A 50-year-old librarian, Mr Y, was arrested for threatening his boss, having been made redundant after 30 years. He had no psychiatric history. Mr Y was convinced that the boss had plotted against him. His diary revealed an increasing preoccupation with these ideas and included allegations and events known to be false. Hallucinations, thought disorder, mood disorder and substance misuse were excluded. Mr Y was single, without close friends, and had a lifelong interest in spying. He reluctantly agreed to take haloperidol, which gradually resolved the delusions and he stopped pestering his ex-boss. However, the beliefs remained in attenuated form, and he continued to suspect various conspiracies were going on.

Specific variants of persistent delusional disorders

The following variants of persistent delusional disorder are mentioned either because of their clinical importance or because they have a memorable eponym and are beloved by examiners.

• *Morbid (pathological) jealousy* is not uncommon and is potentially dangerous. The patient, usually male, has the delusional belief that his partner is unfaithful. He may go to elaborate lengths to prove this and remains unconvinced by evidence to the contrary. He may threaten and finally attack his partner or the alleged third party. Usually morbid jealousy is a

symptom of psychotic depression, schizophrenia or an alcoholic psychosis, but it can be seen in isolation. The risks posed by morbid jealousy (and other psychoses with potentially dangerous delusions or hallucinations) sometimes over-rule patient confidentiality so that the intended victim can be warned (p. 75). Full risk assessment is mandatory.

• *Monosymptomatic hypochondriacal psychosis (somatic delusional disorder)* is the delusional belief that the person has an illness or deformity. It can lead to a prolonged search for inappropriate medical or surgical treatments. It must be distinguished from dysmorphophobia (p. 103).

• In *De Clerambault's syndrome (erotomania)*, the patient, usually female, has a delusion that a man of high standing (a pop star, even a psychiatrist) is in love with her. Some stalkers have this disorder.

• In *folie à deux*, two people, often isolated sisters, share the same delusions. One is genuinely psychotic, the other is 'induced' to become so and is said to recover spontaneously when the two are separated.

• *Capgras' delusion* is the belief that someone close has been replaced by a double. *Fregoli's delusion* is the belief that someone close to them is impersonating other people. Both have been called syndromes, but they are symptoms. They occur in schizophrenia and dementia, and after right-hemisphere damage.

Management and prognosis of delusional disorders

Delusional disorders, like all psychoses, usually respond to antipsychotic drugs.

• Acute delusional disorders often resolve within days, especially if the triggering stressor is removed. Full recovery is the rule although relapses may occur. Some acute psychoses turn out to be the first presentation of schizophrenia or other chronic conditions.

• Persistent delusional disorders can be resistant to treatment (or go untreated) and continue for years. Unlike schizophrenia, negative symptoms rarely occur. It is claimed that pimozide (p. 64) is more effective than other antipsychotics for these conditions, but the evidence is weak.

12.7.3 Schizotypal disorder

The key features of schizotypal disorder are:
• A cold, aloof and suspicious manner.
• Eccentric behaviour.
• Avoidance of social contact.
• Odd beliefs and magical thinking.
• Vague, rambling or metaphorical speech.
• Tendency to odd ideas and sensory experiences.
• At least three of the above present for more than 2 years.

Schizotypal disorder is like a chronic, watered-down version of schizophrenia, in which the odd beliefs stop short of being delusional, and the odd sensory experiences are not quite hallucinatory.
• Schizotypal disorder appears to have a similar genetic background to schizophrenia.
• Schizotypal disorder is diagnosed infrequently, partly because people rarely come into psychiatric contact, and partly because it overlaps with paranoid and schizoid personality disorders (p. 147).
• There are no specific treatments.

12.8 SUMMARY: KEY POINTS

• Schizophrenia is a psychosis characterized by specific types of delusions, hallucinations and thought disorder, called first-rank symptoms. By definition, schizophrenia is not secondary to a mood disorder or an organic disorder and the symptoms must have lasted more than a month.
• Some patients progress to a chronic state where social isolation, apathy and poverty of speech predominate. These are called negative symptoms, in contrast to the positive symptoms which characterize the acute episodes.

• Antipsychotics are effective for positive symptoms but they do not prevent or treat negative symptoms. Clozapine is an atypical antipsychotic which is effective in some otherwise treatment-resistant cases.
• Many patients with schizophrenia need long-term, multidisciplinary support. Psychological and social interventions are an integral part of management.
• Schizophrenia is a neurodevelopmental disorder caused primarily by genetic factors.

CHAPTER 13

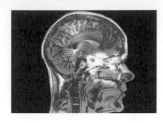

Organic Psychiatric Disorders

Organic psychiatric disorders are those with demonstrable pathological lesions or which arise directly from a medical disorder, in contrast to all other psychiatric disorders which are traditionally called *functional*. This distinction is flawed (p. 1) and causes some problems:

• The major organic disorders, *dementia* and *delirium*, are defined, like other psychiatric syndromes, by their characteristic clinical features. They are caused by various aetiologies and pathologies, which must be identified to make a complete diagnosis.

• Other organic disorders are simply psychiatric disorders *of any type* which appear, in a particular case, to be caused by an identifiable medical disorder. Sometimes it is the psychiatric symptoms which first bring the person to medical attention.

• Psychiatric disorders which are considered *psychological reactions* to illness — such as becoming depressed after being told you have cancer — are excluded from the organic category.

• Substance misuse disorders are organic, in that there is a specific pharmacological cause. By convention they are classified separately (Chapter 14).

13.1 Dementia

13.1.1 Clinical features of dementia

Dementia is also known as *chronic brain syndrome* or *chronic brain failure*. Its cardinal

feature is memory impairment (short-term worse than long-term) in the presence of normal consciousness (cf. delirium). Other features are:

• Symptoms present for 6 months, of sufficient severity to impair functioning.

• Personality and behavioural change, e.g. wandering, aggression, disinhibition.

• Dysphasias, dyspraxias and focal neurological signs may be present.

• Psychotic symptoms (especially visual hallucinations) in half of cases at some stage.

• Unawareness of deficits (except early on).

• Nearly always progressive.

The incidence of dementia rises rapidly with age, affecting < 5% of 65-year-olds and 20% of 80-year-olds. The risk of dementia is doubled in those with an affected first-degree relative. Other risk factors depend on the type of dementia concerned.

• Dementia in the under 65s is termed *presenile dementia*.

• See vignette on p. 78.

13.1.2 Differential diagnosis of dementia

Mild dementia can be confused with several other conditions:

• *Depression.* Poor concentration and impaired memory are common in depression in the elderly — *pseudodementia*. Two questions which help distinguish depression from dementia are:

Did low mood or poor memory come first?

Table 13.1 Causes of dementia.

Alzheimer's disease (~60% of cases)
Vascular dementia (multi-infarct dementia) (~20% of cases)
Lewy body dementia (~15% of cases)
Other causes (<10% of cases)
Degenerative disorders
Pick's disease
Lobar atrophy
Huntington's disease
Prion disease (Creutzfeldt–Jakob disease)
Metabolic disorders
Alcoholic dementia
Vitamin B12 deficiency*
Cerebral anoxia
Normal pressure hydrocephalus*
Infections
HIV*
Syphilis*
Space-occupying lesion
Tumour*
Subdural haematoma*
Head injury

*Potentially treatable causes.

Is the failure to answer questions due to lack of ability or lack of motivation?

Depression and dementia can, of course, occur together.

• *Delirium*. Check level of consciousness and duration of history (p. 18).

• *Deafness*. Check the person can hear.

• *Dysphasia*. Check they can speak.

• *Amnesic syndrome*. A purer short-term memory defect (p. 133).

• *Late-onset schizophrenia (paraphrenia)*. Check for prominent symptoms of psychosis.

13.1.3 The causes of dementia

The common dementias are listed in Table 13.1.

• Alzheimer's disease often coexists with Lewy body dementia.

• In presenile dementia, a higher percentage of cases are due to rare genetic disorders, HIV and head injury.

Clinical features differentiating the dementias

Careful clinical evaluation identifies the specific dementia in > 80% of cases (Table 13.2).

13.1.4 Investigation of dementia

In the history and examination, look for clues pointing towards one of the diagnoses in Table 13.2. For example, a history of a fall (? subdural haematoma) or incontinence (? normal pressure hydrocephalus); on examination you might find hypertension and a carotid bruit (? vascular dementia).

Table 13.3 shows the baseline and specialized tests used in the investigation of dementia. Only the baseline blood tests would routinely be ordered, with further investigation depending on the age of the patient and the suggestion of a treatable aetiology (for example, a CT scan to exclude a subdural haematoma). In the absence of such clues, further tests in an elderly person rarely change the diagnosis, let alone reveal a reversible cause.

• Conversely, in a young person, every effort is made to make a diagnosis — not only in case it is treatable and to inform about prognosis, but also because the dementia may well be inherited and genetic testing available for the family. Presenile dementia is usually referred to neurologists.

13.1.5 Pathology and aetiology of the common dementias

Alzheimer's disease

The cardinal diagnostic features are neurofibrillary tangles and senile (β-amyloid) plaques in the hippocampus and cerebral cortex. Loss of synapses is also important. Neurochemically, the main abnormality is a loss of acetylcholine due to degeneration of the cholinergic neurones of the basal forebrain. The cholinergic deficits and synaptic loss are proportional to the severity of the dementia.

A considerable amount is now known about the aetiology of the disease (Table 13.4):

• The major risk factor is the E4 variant of the apolipoprotein E (apoE) gene. Three polymorphisms exist, apoE2, apoE3 and apoE4

Table 13.2 Clinical features distinguishing between the dementias.

Disease	Prominent symptoms and signs	Other clinical features
Alzheimer's disease	Memory loss, especially short-term Dysphasia and dyspraxia Sense of smell impaired early Persecutory beliefs	Relentlessly progressive Survival 5–10 years
Vascular dementia	Personality change Labile mood Preserved insight	Stepwise progression Signs of vascular disease History of hypertension Commoner in men
Lewy body dementia	Fluctuating dementia Delirium-like phases Parkinsonism Visual hallucinations	Antipsychotics may worsen condition
Pick's disease	Frontal lobe dysfunction Personality change Memory preserved	Slowly progressive Family history Commoner in women

Huntington's disease	Schizophrenia-like psychosis
	Abnormal movements
	    (choreiform)
	Depression and irritability
	Dementia occurs later
		Presents in the 20s–40s
		Strong family history (autosomal
		    dominant)

Normal pressure hydrocephalus	Frontal lobe dysfunction Urinary incontinence Problems walking (gait apraxia)	Commonest in 50–70-year-olds

Prion disease
    (Creutzfeldt–Jakob
    disease)
	Myoclonic jerks
	Seizures
	Cerebellar ataxia
		Often presenile
		Rapid onset and progression
		Death within a year

(the whereabouts of E1 is unknown!). The 15% of the population with one copy of E4 have three times the risk of Alzheimer's disease; the 2% who are E4 homozygotes have a 15-fold greater risk and are highly likely to get the disease if they live to 75.

• The rare early-onset familial cases are due to a mutation in one of three genes — amyloid precursor protein (APP) and presenilin 1 and 2. The β-amyloid found in senile plaques is a fragment of APP.

• The environmental risk factors are of modest effect size.

• The disease process is envisaged as an 'amyloid cascade'. The central event is mis-metabolism of APP to an insoluble form of β-amyloid (Fig. 13.1).

Other dementias

Key elements of other dementias are summarized in Table 13.5.

• *Prion disease* (Creutzfeldt–Jakob disease, CJD) is exceedingly rare but of interest because of the epidemic of bovine spongiform encephalopathy (BSE) — prion disease in cattle — in the UK, and the fact that prion disease is transmissible by diet. As at March 1998, 24 human prion disease cases attributed to BSE have been reported. Unlike typical CJD, these have occurred in young adults and have

Table 13.3 Investigation of dementia.

Test	What the test may show
Blood tests	
Full blood count	Macrocytosis; anaemia
Electrolytes	Hypercalcaemia; renal disease
Liver function tests	Alcoholic liver disease
Thyroid function	Hypothyroidism
Vitamin B12 and folate levels	Deficiencies can produce dementia
Syphilis serology	Formerly common, now rare but overlooked
HIV test	Dementia common in AIDS
Radiography	
Chest X-ray	Bronchial carcinoma with ?cerebral metastases
Brain imaging (CT or MRI)	Tumour; infarcts; haematoma; temporal lobe atrophy suggests Alzheimer's
EEG	Characteristic abnormality in prion disease (3 Hz 'spike and wave')
Other tests	
Lumbar puncture	Normal pressure hydrocephalus; herpes encephalitis
Cerebral blood flow studies	Parietal hypometabolism suggests Alzheimer's
Neuropsychological testing	Assess severity; profile of deficits may point to brain region most affected
Genetic testing	Available for some familial dementias — an area of rapid developments
Brain biopsy	Mainly for suspected prion disease. Rarely performed otherwise

Table 13.4 Causes of Alzheimer's disease.

Factor	Comments
Genetic	
ApoE (chromosome 19)	ApoE4 allele markedly increases risk
Amyloid precursor protein (chromosome 21)	Autosomal dominant mutations which cause early-onset familial Alzheimer's disease
Presenilin 1 (chromosome 14)	
Presenilin 2 (chromosome 1)	
Down's syndrome (trisomy 21)	Alzheimer's disease invariably occurs in middle age
Environmental — risk factors	
Increasing age	Predominant 'risk factor'
Head injury	Doubles risk of Alzheimer's disease
Latent herpes simplex infection	In people with an apoE4 allele
Aluminium exposure	Doubtful
Environmental — protective factors	
Non-steroidal anti-inflammatory drugs	? Retard a possible chronic inflammatory process
Oestrogen replacement therapy (HRT)	? Because oestrogens are neuroprotective
High educational level	'Use it or lose it'
Smoking	Reason controversial

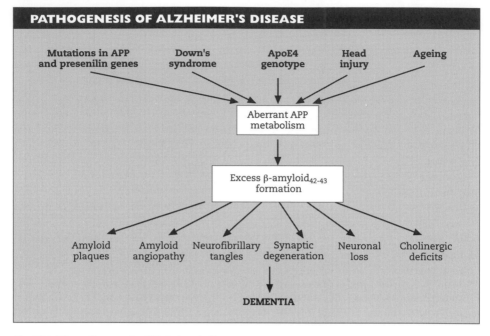

Fig. 13.1 The pathogenesis of Alzheimer's disease.

Table 13.5 Pathology and aetiology of some non-Alzheimer dementias.

Disease	Neuropathology	Aetiology

Vascular dementia	Multiple white matter infarcts
	Dementia proportional to
	    volume infarcted
		Associated with atherosclerosis risk
		    factors

Lewy body dementia	Lewy bodies in cortical neurons Cholinergic deficits	Unknown. ApoE4 may be a risk factor
Pick's disease	Pick bodies in cortical neurons Atrophy of frontotemporal poles Neuronal loss and gliosis	Autosomal dominant. Gene unknown Lobar atrophy is a related condition

Huntington's disease	Atrophy of caudate nucleus
	Loss of spiny neurons in caudate
	Late frontal lobe atrophy
		Autosomal dominant mutations in
		    huntingtin gene
		Mutations are 'triplet repeat
		    expansions'

Prion disease	Aberrant prion protein deposition Spongiform change Neuronal loss and gliosis	Familial cases due to prion gene mutations Iatrogenic Idiopathic

presented (to psychiatrists) with depression and personality change.

13.1.6 Management of dementia

Occasionally, dementia is reversible (see Table 13.1) and responds to appropriate treatment. In most cases, management of dementia has more modest goals, the main one being to optimize quality of life for patient and carer. The following principles and strategies are important:

• Characterize and aim to treat the non-cognitive abnormalities. Simple interventions can improve problems such as wandering (e.g. by organizing regular exercise or raising the door handle) and incontinence (e.g. by a toileting routine). Psychotic symptoms and agitation respond to low-dose antipsychotics (but see below). Treat depression — selective serotonin reuptake inhibitors (SSRIs) are better than tricyclic antidepressants (TCAs) (p. 66).

Fig. 13.2 Pharmacological treatment strategies for Alzheimer's disease.

• Social interventions such as meals-on-wheels, day care and respite admissions help carers cope.
• Sudden deterioration may be due to super-imposed delirium (e.g. due to a urinary tract infection).
• In advanced dementia, palliative rather than active treatment is often indicated. Next-of-kin should be fully involved in these decisions (see vignette, p. 78).

Treatment of Alzheimer's disease

Various agents are being developed which may slow cognitive decline or progression (e.g. time to institutionalization) in Alzheimer's disease (Fig. 13.2). However, the improvements are minor and on current evidence the drugs are not recommended for routine use.

• No drugs are yet available to inhibit the aberrant APP metabolism central to the disease process (Fig. 13.1) but much pharmaceutical research is under way.

13.1.7 Prognosis of dementia

Most dementias progress inexorably. Death is usually within 10 years of onset, with some dementias progressing much more rapidly

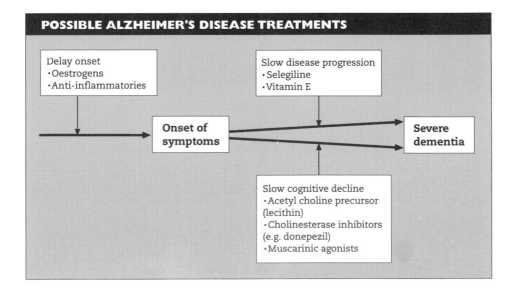

(Table 13.2). Younger cases and those with focal neurological signs or psychotic symptoms have a worse prognosis.

• People with dementia should not be donors in view of the risk of transmission of prion disease.

13.2 Delirium

Delirium is also known as *acute confusional state* or *acute brain syndrome*. It is common on medical and surgical wards — a third of elderly patients in hospital have an episode of delirium — so all doctors should be able to recognize and manage it.

13.2.1 Clinical features of delirium
Clouding of consciousness (p. 13) is the most important diagnostic sign. It is manifested as drowsiness, decreased awareness of surroundings, disorientation in time and place and distractibility. At its most severe the patient may be unresponsive (p. 33), but more commonly the impaired consciousness is quite subtle. Indeed the first clue to the presence of delirium is often one of its other features:
• Visual hallucinations.
• Transient persecutory delusions.
• Irritability, sometimes aggression.
• Impaired concentration and memory.
• Fluctuating course, worse at night.

13.2.2 Aetiology of delirium
Recognition of delirium should be followed by an urgent search for its cause (Table 13.6).

13.2.3 Management of delirium
Delirium is managed where it occurs — usually in general hospitals. Psychiatrists may be asked to assess the patient, make the diagnosis and give advice. Treatment is directed at both the symptoms and the cause, and includes both medical and nursing interventions (Table 13.7).

13.2.4 Prognosis of delirium
Prognosis depends on the cause. Within a week the patient is usually better or has died.

Table 13.6 Common causes of delirium.

Drugs
Alcohol intoxication
Alcohol withdrawal and delirium tremens
Opiates
Prescribed drugs
Any drug with anticholinergic properties
Any sedative
Digoxin
Diuretics
Lithium
Steroids
Medical conditions
Febrile illness
Septicaemia
Organ failure (cardiac, renal, hepatic)
Hypoglycaemia
Postoperative hypoxia
Neurological conditions
Epileptic seizure (postictal)
Head injury
Space-occupying lesion
Encephalitis

Table 13.7 Management of delirium.

Medical components
Investigate and treat underlying cause (e.g. give antibiotics, oxygen; stop incriminated drug)
Monitor vital signs
Control agitation or psychotic symptoms
Low-dose antipsychotics (benzodiazepines if delirium tremens)
Nursing components
Quiet surroundings (sideroom), constant lighting
Regular routine (to reduce disorientation and agitation)

The 3-month mortality is 25%. There is no good evidence that delirium progresses to dementia.

A 75-year-old lady is found lying on the floor and is brought into casualty. She is disorientated in time and place, distractible, and unable to give any history. She thinks you are trying to kill her. She is febrile, tachycardic and hypotensive, but has no neurological signs or injuries. Blood tests and X-rays are performed. She is admitted, and given oxygen and antibiotics for the clinical suspicion of septicaemia. Her agitation worsens but settles with haloperidol. The GP tells you that there is no past history of note. Blood cultures grow an organism which is sensitive to the antibiotic. Her condition improves over 48 hours. The haloperidol is tailed off and cognitive testing a week later is normal.

13.3 Other organic disorders

Dementia and delirium have been described in detail because they are common. As mentioned at the start of the chapter, there are many other organic conditions which can present together with the whole range of psychiatric disorders. The important principles, and some specific examples, are summarized here.

13.3.1 Organic psychiatric disorders

The diagnostic rule is to preface the psychiatric label with 'organic' and to state the aetiology (Table 13.8). For example, 'organic anxiety disorder due to thyrotoxicosis'.

Each organic syndrome is very rare compared to its 'functional' counterpart. Indeed, in areas with good primary care, psychiatrists rarely see undiagnosed organic psychiatric disorders. However, when an organic syndrome does occur it is essential to recognize it —

always include the possibility in a case presentation or psychiatric examination. Detecting an organic disorder requires that you:
• Always consider the possibility. If this is done, it is easier not to forget to take a brief medical history and conduct a relevant physical examination (p. 14).
• Are suspicious if aspects of the psychiatric presentation are unusual. For example, organic syndromes often produce abnormalities in unexpected functions, e.g. anosmia in depression due to a frontal meningioma.

There may or may not be an effective treatment for the organic disorder. Regardless, the psychiatric symptoms are still treated with appropriate pharmacological, psychological and social interventions.

13.3.2 Amnesic syndrome

Amnesic (or *amnestic*) syndrome completes the triad of conditions (with dementia and delirium) which affect memory and which always have an organic cause. Its features are:
• Selective loss of recent memory.
• *Confabulation* — the unconscious fabrication of recent events to cover gaps in memory.
• Time disorientation.
• Attention and immediate recall intact.
• Long-term memory and other intellectual faculties preserved.

Amnesic syndrome is rare. It is due to damage to the mammillary bodies, hippocampus or thalamus. The usual cause is alcohol-induced thiamine deficiency (*Korsakov's syndrome*). Treat with thiamine and abstinence. The deficits are often irreversible.

Table 13.8 Organic psychiatric disorders.

Syndrome	Example of cause
Organic brain syndromes	Dementia, delirium, amnesic syndrome
Organic delusional (psychotic) disorders	Systemic lupus erythematosus
Organic mood disorders	Multiple sclerosis
Organic anxiety disorders	Thyrotoxicosis
Organic personality disorders	After head injury

13.3.3 Epilepsy

Epilepsy sits on the bridge between psychiatry and neurology. It is a common, heterogeneous disorder (Table 13.9). Detailed descriptions are found in neurology texts. Here we examine the psychiatric implications of epilepsy (Table 13.10).

Relationship of psychiatric symptoms and seizures

Complex partial epilepsy was formerly called *psychomotor epilepsy* because of the frequency of psychiatric symptoms during seizures (Table 13.11). Psychiatric presentations are rarer with the other forms of epilepsy. *Absence seizures* in children produce transient lapses in concentration or simple automatisms and can be mistaken for a behavioural disorder. A *generalized seizure* can present to a psychiatrist if, for example, the person is found wandering in a postictal delirium.

- A *pseudoseizure* is a form of dissociative disorder (p. 101). It can be distinguished from a true seizure clinically (lack of incontinence or self-injury), by EEG monitoring, or by plasma prolactin, which is raised by a genuine seizure.
- Other conditions which can be misdiagnosed as epilepsy include schizophrenia, panic attacks

Table 13.9 The epilepsies.

Type	Other names	Comments	Conscious level during seizure
Generalized seizures		No focal onset	
Tonic–clonic	Grand mal	The classic type of seizure	Unconscious
Absence	Petit mal	Subtle and brief	Impaired
Miscellaneous		Myoclonic or atonic	Variable
Partial seizures		Focal onset	
Simple partial			Unaffected
Complex partial	Psychomotor, temporal lobe epilepsy (TLE)	Of most psychiatric significance	Impaired

Table 13.10 Psychiatric aspects of epilepsy.

Category	Example
Psychiatric symptoms related to seizures	
Due to shared aetiology	Temporal lobe tumour
At start of seizure	Hallucinations during aura
During seizure	Non-convulsive status presenting as fugue (p. 102)
After seizure	Postictal delirium
Between seizures	Psychosis of complex partial epilepsy
Psychiatric disorder masquerading as epilepsy	Pseudoseizures
Psychiatric disorder associated with epilepsy	
Depression	Common in people with epilepsy
Suicide	Several times more common in people with epilepsy
Psychiatric problems of treatment	
Side-effects of anticonvulsants	Depression with barbiturates
Seizures as medication side-effect	Antipsychotics and tricyclic antidepressants

Table 13.11 Psychiatric symptoms of complex partial seizures.

During the seizure (ictal)
Impaired consciousness
Hallucinations and distorted perceptions
Olfactory
Bodily — especially epigastric
Sense of *déjà vu*
Depersonalization and derealization
Speech and memory affected
Automatisms and stereotyped behaviour
Between seizures (interictal)
Schizophrenia-like psychosis (especially if
seizure focus in left temporal lobe)
Depression
Sexual dysfunction and lack of libido

and hypoglycaemia. In children, consider temper tantrums and nightmares.

Psychological problems associated with having epilepsy

Historically, epilepsy was attributed to demonic possession and its sufferers were seen as irritable, self-centred people with criminal tendencies. Although these ideas are entirely false, persisting negative attitudes, together with the real disabilities, explain the higher incidence of neurosis, mood disorder and suicide in epilepsy.

• Anticonvulsant treatments can compound the problems — phenobarbitone causes hyperactivity and irritability in children; phenytoin can produce ataxia and delirium.

13.3.4 Head injury

Head injury is a major cause of organic psychiatric syndromes in young adults. These syndromes can be difficult to treat and services are under-resourced.

• The psychiatric consequences of a head injury depend partly on the nature and location of the injury, and partly on the person's premorbid characteristics. In blunt trauma, the brain suffers contusions at the point of impact,

focal damage elsewhere as the brain reverberates in the skull, and diffuse axonal damage due to the shearing forces. People with an apoE4 allele (p. 127) are at greater risk of dying after head injury and of being left with persistent deficits if they survive.

Cognitive impairment after head injury

A head injury with loss of consciousness may produce amnesia, either *anterograde* (post-traumatic), for events after the injury, or *retrograde*. Anterograde amnesia for a period > 24 hours predicts a poor long-term outcome, including persistent cognitive deficits.

• The impairment ranges from a subtle slowing of thought and distractibility through to dementia.

• It tends to improve in the first year but thereafter deficits are likely to be permanent. There is no specific treatment.

Other psychiatric consequences of head injury

• *Personality changes* are frequent. Typically the changes are indicative of frontal lobe damage: impaired ability to plan or persevere; emotional shallowness and lability; impulsivity and irritability. Altered sexual behaviour (in any direction) and long-winded speech also occur. Improvement is partial and slow.

• *Mood disorder, anxiety disorders* and *schizophrenia* are commoner than expected after head injury. Left- and right-sided frontal lobe damage are associated with depression and mania, respectively.

• *Postconcussional syndrome* describes emotional, cognitive and bodily symptoms occurring after relatively minor head injury. The symptoms are sometimes thought to be 'psychological' or even feigned, related to hopes of compensation. There is little evidence for this belief.

13.3.5 Other medical disorders associated with psychiatric disorders

Table 13.12 lists some medical disorders which often have psychiatric manifestations.

Table 13.12 Medical disorders with psychiatric manifestations.

Medical disorder	Psychiatric manifestations
Cerebral tumour	Psychiatric symptoms in 50%, more so if tumour is in frontal or temporal lobes
Cerebral abscess	May present with psychiatric symptoms
Multiple sclerosis	Mood disturbance in 25% — euphoria or depression. Cognitive deficits in 25%. Personality changes in 25% — apathy, irritability
HIV	Dementia in 30% with AIDS. Psychosis — prevalence uncertain
Systemic lupus erythematosus (SLE)	5% at presentation; 50% at some stage — mood disorder, psychosis, delirium, seizures
Cushing's disease	Severe depression common. Occasionally psychosis and cognitive impairment. (Mania more usual when steroids given therapeutically)
Addison's disease	Apathy and fatigue in 80%; depression in 50%; cognitive impairments in 50%; psychosis in 5%
Hyperthyroidism	Anxiety (common), depression, mania, delirium
Hypothyroidism	Mental slowing and depressive symptoms very common. Rarely 'myxoedema madness' — delirium, depression, dementia. Symptoms may persist despite thyroxine replacement
Hypercalcaemia	Psychosis, delirium and mood disorders in 50%; cognitive impairment in 25%

13.4 SUMMARY: KEY POINTS

• Organic psychiatric disorders are those due to a recognized medical cause or pathology.

• Dementia and delirium are by definition organic disorders; all other psychiatric disorders *can* be. Hence consider an organic cause for every psychiatric presentation — epilepsy and endocrine disorders are classic culprits.

• Dementia is characterized by impaired memory. It is usually gradual in onset, progressive and untreatable. The commonest cause is Alzheimer's disease.

• Delirium is acute cognitive impairment secondary to clouding of consciousness. It has many causes (e.g. drugs, septicaemia). It is usually treatable but has a significant mortality.

• Treatment of organic disorders is aimed at the underlying cause *and* at the psychiatric symptoms.

CHAPTER 14

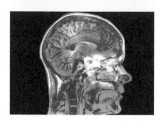

Substance Misuse

14.1 General issues

Many substances are taken for pleasure. A substance is *misused* if it produces physical, psychological or social harm. Commonly misused substances are shown in Table 14.1. This chapter describes:
- the features of substance misuse;
- the psychiatric consequences; and
- the management of substance misuse and its associated psychiatric disorders.

Substance misuse presents in diverse ways. For example: as depression or morbid jealousy

Table 14.1 Commonly misused substances.

Alcohol
Cannabis
Opioids
Heroin
Morphine
Methadone
Stimulants
Amphetamines
Cocaine
3,4-methylenedioxymethamphetamine
(MDMA, ecstasy)
Hallucinogens
Lysergic acid diethylamide (LSD)
Phencyclidine (PCP)
Solvents
Legal substances
Benzodiazepines
Nicotine
Caffeine

(both associated with alcohol); as an acute psychosis (amphetamines); or as haematemesis (alcoholic cirrhosis).
- Review the substance misuse module (p. 31).

There are no reliable prevalence figures for misuse of substances other than alcohol (p. 139), since honesty about an illegal activity is unlikely. It is clear that clinic data or statistics about registered addicts give a misleading impression of what substances are being misused and what their common health consequences are. Bear this in mind when reading sections 14.3–14.7.
- In the USA, 1.5% of adults admit to having tried heroin, 7% amphetamines, 8% LSD, 12% cocaine and 30% cannabis. A quarter of each group were regular users.

14.1.1 Types of substance misuse

There are several categories of substance misuse:
- *At-risk consumption.* (Alcohol) intake at a level associated with increased risk of harm.
- *Harmful use.* Misuse associated with health and social consequences, but without dependence.
- *Dependence.* Prolonged, regular use of some substances (especially alcohol, opioids, amphetamines) can lead to *dependence* (*addiction*) and *withdrawal* syndromes.

Intoxication is the acute effect of the substance — being drunk (alcohol), tripping (LSD) or stoned (cannabis).

• Intoxication with illicit drugs may lead to a psychiatric presentation (e.g. as an acute psychosis).

14.1.2 Assessment and management of substance misuse

Assessment

The principles of assessment are similar for all substances:

• Be willing and able to ask screening questions (p. 10).

• Know the features of misuse of alcohol and other commonly used substances.

• Be aware of the psychiatric and medical disorders associated with substance misuse.

In acute situations, testing for the drug is useful. Alcohol can be measured in breath or blood; most illicit drugs or their metabolites can be detected in the urine — some briefly (e.g. amphetamines), some for weeks afterwards (cannabis).

Management

Management is also based upon a set of uniform principles:

• Identify at-risk consumption and harmful use early, and give accurate information and advice.

• In dependency, facilitate withdrawal (detoxification). If impossible, minimize harm associated with continuing use.

• Treat complications. For example, drug-induced psychosis secondary to amphetamines; septicaemia in an intravenous drug user.

• Help maintain abstinence following withdrawal — a form of rehabilitation.

• Prevention — this largely involves population-level interventions such as pricing policies.

To achieve these goals, a variety of psychological, pharmacological and social treatment methods are used. See below, and vignette on p. 79.

14.1.3 The aetiology of substance misuse

Substance misuse has a multifactorial aetiology (Table 14.2). Together, the factors determine both the prevalence and the type of substance misused.

• Aetiology has been studied in most detail for alcohol. Similar factors confer vulnerability to misuse of substances in general (and perhaps to other addictions such as gambling).

Table 14.2 Factors associated with substance misuse.

Genetic
    Variation in metabolizing enzymes
    Variation in occurrence of withdrawal phenomena
    Variation in dopamine receptor and transporter genes
Neurobiological
    Brain activity: trait differences in EEG patterns
    Chemicals: abnormalities in dopamine, GABA, endogenous opioids and their receptors
    Anatomical: key site is nucleus accumbens
Psychological
    Personality factors
    Learned behaviour
    Positive reinforcement — the drugs lead to behaviours which increase their use
Socioeconomic
    Price and availability
    Cultural norms and acceptability
Legal
    Restrictions on sale
    Penalties for possession or dealing

14.2 Alcohol

14.2.1 Definitions and epidemiology

Most adults drink alcohol, and many drink too much — 27% of men and 11% of women drink more than the recommended limits (21 and 14 units/week for men and women, respectively). Seven per cent of men and 2% of women are dependent on alcohol (Fig. 14.1).

• Consumption of alcohol by teenagers is increasing — 12% of 11–15-year-olds are regular drinkers.

At levels below the recommended limit, alcohol consumption is associated with lower mortality rates than in teetotallers. As intake exceeds the limits, however, there is an escalating morbidity and mortality (Table 14.3).

• Alcohol causes 28 000 deaths/year in the UK, including 3000 from alcohol poisoning and cirrhosis.

• Thirty per cent of drivers killed in road accidents are above the legal limit for blood alcohol.

14.2.2 Clinical features of alcohol misuse

Dependence

The concept of dependence was introduced on p. 32. Diagnosis of alcohol dependence (*alcoholism*) needs three or more of the following:

• Feeling compelled to drink.

• Primacy of drinking over other activities such as eating, family life, work, health.

• Increased tolerance to alcohol — being able to drink quantities that would incapacitate others.

• Relief drinking — drinking to stop or prevent withdrawal symptoms.

• Stereotyped pattern of drinking.

• Reinstatement after abstinence — unable to give up alcohol for long.

• Drinking despite awareness of harmful consequences.

• Withdrawal symptoms.

Withdrawal and delirium tremens

The main features of alcohol withdrawal are:

• tremulousness ('the shakes');

• agitation;

• nausea and retching;

• sweating; and

• overwhelming desire to drink (craving).

Withdrawal symptoms are relieved by alcohol — hence the CAGE eye-opener question (p. 10). If untreated the symptoms may last for several days. Transient misperceptions and hallucinations may occur — objects appear distorted and shadows seem to move; disorganized voices or snatches of music may be heard.

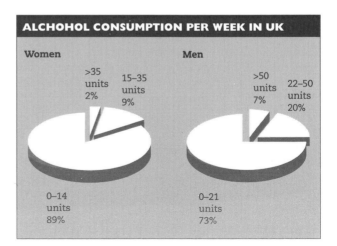

ALCHOHOL CONSUMPTION PER WEEK IN UK

Women

>35 units 2%
15–35 units 9%
0–14 units 89%

Men

>50 units 7%
22–50 units 20%
0–21 units 73%

Fig. 14.1 Weekly consumption of alcohol in adults in UK. One unit is 13.5 g alcohol. Dependence is likely if regular intake exceeds 50 units per week in men and 35 in women.

Table 14.3 Harmful effects of alcohol.

Medical
Liver damage — hepatitis, cirrhosis
Cardiovascular — cardiomyopathy,
    hypertension
Gastrointestinal — peptic ulcer, oesophageal
    varices, pancreatitis
Neoplasms — liver, oesophagus
Blood — anaemia, haemochromatosis

Neurological and neuropsychiatric
Blackouts
Epilepsy
Neuropathy
Delirium tremens
Wernicke's syndrome
Korsakov's syndrome
Cerebellar degeneration
Central pontine myelinosis
Head injury (from falls)

Psychiatric
Alcoholic hallucinosis
Morbid jealousy
Alcoholic dementia
Depressive disorders
Anxiety disorders
Sexual dysfunction
Suicide

Social
Accidents
Problems with relationships
Domestic violence
Employment difficulties
Crime

• Withdrawal symptoms often occur on waking as the blood alcohol concentration falls during sleep.

The most severe form of withdrawal (5% of cases) is *delirium tremens* (the 'DTs'), a potentially fatal condition. Its characteristics are:
• onset 24–48 hours after stopping heavy, prolonged drinking;
• delirium (clouding of consciousness, disorientation);
• visual hallucinations;
• delusions, usually persecutory and transient misidentification of people around the patient;
• fear and agitation, sometimes aggression;
• coarse tremor;
• seizures;
• autonomic disturbance (sweating, fever, tachycardia, hypertension);
• insomnia; and
• dehydration and electrolyte disturbance.
Delirium tremens lasts 3–4 days, followed by exhaustion and patchy amnesia for the episode.

Wernicke's syndrome
An acute encephalopathy presenting with delirium, ataxia, nystagmus and ophthalmoplegia, occurring in the severely alcohol dependent, usually in the context of withdrawal. It is due to thiamine deficiency and requires urgent treatment. It may progress to Korsakov's syndrome (p. 133).

Harmful alcohol use
There are no specific features of harmful alcohol use, since it is defined as people who have problems due to alcohol intake but who are not dependent. It may be detected in several ways; for example:
• on inquiry in any medical setting;
• when a patient volunteers that he thinks he is drinking too much;
• through unexplained macrocytosis or abnormal liver function tests; or
• because of one of its psychiatric or social consequences (Table 14.3).

Associated medical disorders
If alcohol misuse has led to a medical disorder, then psychiatric or social impairments (Table 14.3) are also likely. These should be screened for and appropriate action taken. Conversely, if an alcohol-related psychiatric disorder is diagnosed, check for physical symptoms and signs of alcohol dependency.
• 10% of hospital admissions are for disorders caused by alcohol, and twice that number have significant alcohol-related problems (p. 170).

Associated psychiatric disorders
Alcohol misuse is associated with an increased

risk of, and worse prognosis for, most psychiatric disorders (Table 14.3).

• In *alcoholic hallucinosis*, a heavy drinker experiences recurrent auditory hallucinations, usually of a threatening or derogatory nature. The hallucinations occur in clear consciousness (cf. withdrawal hallucinations). The syndrome is an example of a drug-induced psychosis.

• About 10% of people who are alcohol dependent commit suicide.

14.2.3 Management of alcohol problems

The focus in this section is on clinical, rather than population-based, interventions.

Detection and diagnosis

Detection of alcohol misuse follows the principles outlined on p. 37, and the practical issues covered in the core assessment (p. 10) and substance misuse module (p. 31).

Management of at-risk consumption and harmful alcohol use

A brief intervention in primary care is usually sufficient if someone is drinking more than the safe limits but is not dependent and has no specific medical or psychiatric disorder. The components are:

• Assess accurately the amount consumed (use diaries, informants).

• Assess the nature and extent of harm (e.g. liver function tests, work record).

• Ensure person is fully informed of the hazards of excess alcohol and the benefits of moderation. Tailor advice to individual patients; written information reinforces verbal messages.

• Review progress. If problem drinking persists, give details of further resources available locally.

Treatment of alcohol dependence

The first requirement is detoxification ('detox', 'drying out'), which is controlled withdrawal. It involves a reducing course of a benzodiazepine in place of alcohol. This can usually be under-

taken in primary care, but involve the local substance misuse service and consider admission if the problem is complicated (e.g. comorbid psychiatric disorder, lack of support at home).

• A suggested regimen is chlordiazepoxide, starting at 20 mg qds and reducing daily to finish with 10 mg on day 7. Advise the patient to drink plenty of non-alcoholic liquids. Prescribe vitamins — nutritional deficiencies are common and withdrawal may precipitate Wernicke's syndrome.

• A similar strategy can be used if a patient presents in the early stages of unintentional withdrawal.

• Chlormethiazole (Heminevrin) is no longer recommended due to toxicity and misuse.

Maintaining abstinence

Various strategies are used to prevent relapse following withdrawal from alcohol. None has been shown to be very effective.

• Aim for abstinence — it has a better long-term outcome than controlled drinking.

• Regular liver function tests and breath alcohol measurements help monitor progress.

• Encourage attendance at groups run by local community alcohol services or Alcoholics Anonymous.

• Disulfiram (Antabuse) interacts with alcohol to produce nausea, flushing and choking sensations. It has its own side-effects and requires considerable motivation. Other pharmacological agents to promote abstinence (e.g. acamprosate, opioid antagonists) are currently under evaluation.

• Detoxified drinkers used to be given inpatient psychodynamic psychotherapy. Current psychological interventions include cognitive behavioural therapy, social skills training, problem solving and motivational interviewing (helping them make the decision to change their behaviour).

• Half of those detoxified resume heavy drinking.

Treatment of medical disorders associated with alcohol misuse

Many of the medical syndromes arising from

alcohol misuse can present as emergencies (e.g. Wernicke's encephalopathy, bleeding varices), and the admission provides an opportunity for psychiatric intervention. Look out for withdrawal symptoms occurring during hospitalization.

Treatment of psychiatric disorders associated with alcohol misuse

The principles are:
* To reduce intake to safe limits, since continuing alcohol misuse acts as a perpetuating factor.
* To treat the psychiatric disorder on its merits. Check for interaction of alcohol with prescribed medication, and note that alcohol misuse can prevent psychological treatments being effective.

14.3 Opioids

Opioids (*opiates*) cause high levels of morbidity and mortality, and are very addictive. Heroin is the most common; others include morphine, buprenorphine, codeine and methadone. There are several modes of use:
* *Intravenous injection* ('mainlining'). It is associated with a high risk of infections, thrombosis and phlebitis. Hepatitis B and C and HIV should be suspected and testing performed (with informed consent and appropriate counselling) in anyone who has injected drugs.
* *Inhalation* ('chasing the dragon'). The opiate is melted on metal foil and then inhaled as it vaporizes.
* *'Snorting'*. The opioid is 'cut' into a fine powder and then sniffed.

There are probably around 100 000 regular users in UK.
* The Home Office registration system has been replaced with regional databases.

14.3.1 Clinical features

Dependence

The main effect of opioids is a feeling of euphoria and analgesia. Less pleasant features occurring in regular users include chronic malaise, anorexia, loss of libido, impotence, pinpoint pupils and constipation. Tolerance to all opioids rapidly develops. Because of this (and because of batch-to-batch variation in purity), overdose is common and frequently fatal due to respiratory depression.
* Tolerance makes pain management in an opioid user difficult.

Withdrawal

Stopping opioids leads to an extremely unpleasant withdrawal syndrome ('cold turkey') involving:
* craving;
* restlessness and insomnia;
* myalgia;
* sweating;
* abdominal pain, vomiting and diarrhoea;
* dilated pupils, running nose and eyes;
* tachycardia;
* yawning; and
* 'goose bumps'.

The onset is usually within 8–12 hours of the last dose (longer after methadone), peaking 24–48 hours later and subsiding over 10 days.
* Though symptoms are severe, opioid withdrawal is rarely life-threatening.

14.3.2 Management of opioid dependence

Opioid dependence can be managed in two ways.

Rapid detoxification and abstinence

Inpatient detoxification is more effective than outpatient detoxifixation — probably because opioid-dependent people live in chaotic, unsupportive environments (often with other users).
* Information is given about the nature and course of withdrawal symptoms.
* The patient is prescribed reducing doses of a substitute drug, methadone linctus, which reduces the severity of the withdrawal symptoms. Clonidine and naltrexone (an opioid antagonist) are also used.

Post-withdrawal abstinence programmes vary from specific relapse-prevention therapies to residential houses where a network of ex-users helps the recovering addict overcome the craving.

• Even when withdrawal is achieved, the relapse rate is high (40% at 6 months; most at a year).

Harm reduction and maintenance therapy (substitution treatment)

The AIDS epidemic led to an expansion of maintenance therapy for opioid dependence, with the priority changing from abstinence to 'intermediate goals', i.e. reducing the harm resulting from opioid use.

The first aim of the harm reduction approach is to make services more acceptable to users and so to engage more people in treatment. Then, the aims are to:

• reduce injecting;
• stabilize drug use and lifestyle;
• reduce criminal behaviour by avoiding need to obtain expensive drugs; and
• reduce death rate.

The harm reduction approach is pragmatic and includes a range of initiatives such as the provision of free needles and syringes and public education. A central feature is *substitute prescribing*. Oral methadone is prescribed to prevent the need for intravenous injections. Long-term use of the oral drug is usual.

• Substitute prescribing is not for all opioid users, but should be targeted at those whose social functioning and health have already been seriously affected by their drug use (and where abstinence is an unrealistic goal).

14.4 Stimulants

14.4.1 Amphetamines

Amphetamines ('speed', 'whizz') may be taken orally, snorted or injected. They produce symptoms similar to those of hypomania (p. 85): elevated mood, over-talkativeness, increased energy and insomnia. Pulse and blood pressure increase, pupils dilate and mucous membranes become dry.

• *Dependence* occurs. Regular users develop mood swings. The withdrawal syndrome can be severe (a 'crash'), with agitated depression, lethargy, suicidal thoughts and craving.

• Management and prognosis is similar to that for opioids. Treat intoxication or psychosis with benzodiazepines and antipsychotics; treat depression with tricyclic antidepressants.

• Prolonged use can lead to *paranoid psychosis*. This can continue for months after use has ceased.

• Amphetamines are used clinically for hyperkinetic disorder (p. 158) and narcolepsy (p. 110).

• Amphetamines are potent dopamine enhancers — they stimulate its release and inhibit its reuptake.

14.4.2 Cocaine

Cocaine produces similar effects to amphetamines, but the features tend to be more dramatic.

• Cocaine is either snorted, or smoked in the form of 'crack' or 'freebase' (cocaine processed to remove the hydrochloride), which increases the intensity of the effect.

• Despite its bad reputation, cocaine is no more addictive than amphetamines — perhaps less so.

14.4.3 3,4-Methylenedioxymethamphetamine (MDMA, Ecstasy)

Ecstasy is a synthetic amphetamine analogue with the alerting actions of amphetamines and some hallucinogenic effects (because of a 5-HT-releasing action). It has become widely used in UK — 30% of teenagers say they've tried it — especially in the club culture. Tolerance occurs and the best experience is said to be the first. Though it is safer than amphetamine or cocaine, there is concern about its harmful effects:

• Adverse reactions are — hyperpyrexia and acute renal failure due to dehydration, as well as water intoxication in users who overcompensate. There are rare but well-publicized fatalities.

• Acute psychosis can occur. Prevalence is unknown.
• The drug is neurotoxic to 5-HT fibres and chronic users have lowered central 5-HT levels. There is therefore concern that depression and impulsivity may be long-term consequences of ecstasy use.

14.5 Hallucinogens

Hallucinogens alter perception, producing psychedelic experiences. They are taken orally. LSD is the main synthetic hallucinogen; similar effects can be achieved using magic mushrooms. Agonism at $5\text{-}HT_2$ receptors is a likely common mechanism.

14.5.1 Lysergic acid diethylamide (LSD)
The 'trip' starts about 2 hours after consumption, lasts 8–12 hours, and consists of distorted sensory perception, alteration of the sense of time and scale, and changes in body image (e.g. out-of-body experiences). The effects can be very intense — and occasionally terrifying (a 'bad trip').
• Hallucinogens rarely cause dependence or withdrawal. They are associated with *flashbacks* in which the sensations of a trip are re-experienced long afterwards.
• Emergency psychiatric referral may occur because of the panic or agitation associated with a bad trip. Reassurance, reorientation and 'talking down' are necessary. Sedation can be given as required with benzodiazepines. The person may also come to harm from responding to the hallucinations.

14.6 Cannabis

Cannabis is the most widely used illicit drug. It is derived from the hemp plant *Cannabis sativa*. The main active ingredient is δ-1-tetrahydrocannabinol, which acts on endogenous cannabinoid receptors. Cannabis is usually smoked. It causes several effects including:

• exaggeration of pre-existing mood;
• mellowness and increased enjoyment of aesthetic experience;
• distortion of sense of space and time;
• reddening of eyes; and
• impairment of motor performance — for example, car driving.

Adverse reactions include anxiety and paranoid ideation — especially in first-time users — and occasionally delirium. Cannabis does not cause dependence or withdrawal, though some tolerance occurs (and use may become so ingrained as to warrant the term 'psychological dependence'). Users rarely seek treatment or come to medical attention.
• The occurrence of an 'amotivational state' in chronic heavy users remains unproven.
• Cannabis may be a risk factor for schizophrenia and associated with a worse treatment response.

14.7 Other substances

14.7.1 Phencyclidine
Phencyclidine (PCP, 'angel dust') and ketamine are anaesthetics which, in smaller doses, produce hallucinations, disorientation and agitation. The picture resembles schizophrenia. Complications include nystagmus, tachycardia and seizures.
• Usage is common in the USA but rare in the UK.
• The drugs are antagonists at NMDA glutamate receptors.
• When managing PCP intoxication, avoid chlorpromazine.

14.7.2 Solvents
Solvent misuse (of glue, aerosols, petrol, etc.) is mainly an adolescent male group activity. The effects are rapid in onset and short-lived — euphoria, disinhibition, blurred vision, ataxia.
• Solvent use comes to medical attention when complications arise — cardiac dysrhythmias, inhalation of vomit, coma. Chronic damage to the central nervous system and other organs can occur.

14.7.3 Anabolic steroids

Anabolic steroids are misused mainly by male athletes and bodybuilders. They produce a range of psychiatric effects which can be severe and persistent — euphoria, depression, aggression ('roid rage') and hyperactivity. A form of dependency may result in some users. Clinical suspicion may be aroused by the physical appearance.

14.7.4 Benzodiazepines

Benzodiazepines are taken illicitly, often as part of multiple drug misuse and as an opioid substitute. It can be difficult to decide whether symptoms and side-effects are attributable to the benzodiazepine or to the other drugs being used.

• Benzodiazepine dependence and the man-agement of iatrogenic cases were mentioned on p. 62.

14.7.5 Nicotine and caffeine

Both nicotine and caffeine are addictive — ask any smoker or serious coffee drinker. Each has its own acute actions and side-effects, but psychiatric problems are rare.

• Psychiatric patients smoke more than the population average. Ninety per cent of people with schizophrenia do so (perhaps because nicotine reduces medication side-effects). For unknown reasons they have a much lower incidence of lung cancer than other smokers.

• Abstinence rates after nicotine dependence (30% at 6 months) are worse than for opioids, cocaine and alcohol.

14.8 SUMMARY: KEY POINTS

• For each substance consider:
What are its acute effects?
Does it cause dependence and withdrawal? What are the features?
What are the associated psychiatric, medical and social complications?

• Dependence is a combination of physical and psychological effects in people who regularly use alcohol, opioids or stimulants. Withdrawal occurs if the substance is withheld.

• Substance misuse is widespread. Those in treatment are a small and unrepresentative fraction.

• Alcohol produces a wide range of psychiatric, medical and social problems. In every patient enquire about alcohol intake and consider a role for alcohol misuse in their disorder.

• Management of substance misuse includes psychological, pharmacological and social components. The prognosis for persistent abstinence after being dependent on any substance is poor.

CHAPTER 15

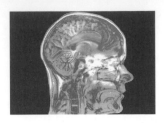

Personality Disorders

15.1 Personality and personality disorder

Personality describes the characteristic behavioural, emotional and cognitive attributes of an individual. Thus we talk about an aggressive man, a nervous lady, an obsessional workaholic, and so on. Such traits are usually apparent by mid-adolescence and remain fairly stable thereafter.

Psychiatrists are interested in personality because it forms part of the contextual understanding of every case (p. 14) and because it interacts with psychiatric disorders (p. 150). Furthermore, psychiatrists see many people with extreme personality traits which cause distress and may be a focus of treatment in their own right. For example:
• a spinster so timid that she has never had a close relationship;
• a tax inspector whose need for tidiness in his office has led to an industrial dispute;
• a housewife whose response to family arguments is to hurl the crockery around.

Personality traits which are excessive and dysfunctional constitute *personality disorder*. People with personality disorder come into contact with medical and psychiatric services either because they are concerned about themselves, or because their actions affect others around them. For example:

• the spinster takes an overdose because she is so lonely;
• the tax inspector's solicitor requests a psychiatric report in his defence;
• the housewife's son is taken to casualty after a plate hits him.

15.2 Clinical features of personality disorders

15.2.1 General features

Personality disorder has a number of characteristics. All should be present before the term is applied:
• A marked deviation of one or more aspects of personality:
    cognitions (attitudes; ways in which people's actions are interpreted);
    mood (range, intensity and appropriateness of emotions);
    impulse control and gratification of needs;
    relationships and the way interpersonal situations are handled.
• Behaviour maladaptive across a range of situations (i.e. not situation-specific).
• The personality attributes cause distress to the individual or those he interacts with.
• The characteristics are pervasive, stable and recognizable from late adolescence onwards.

The diagnosis of personality disorder requires evidence of long-standing emotional or behavioural abnormalities which are not attributable to a psychiatric disorder.
• This requires considerable information about the patient's previous behaviour, personal history and mental state.

15.2.2 The types of personality disorder: categories and clusters

Personality disorder is divided into 10 ICD-10 categories (Table 15.1). However, their validity and reliability are either poor or unknown. Most patients seem to fit either several categories or none of them. A simpler, more evidence-based option (from DSM-IV) is to use three *clusters*:
• *Cluster A: eccentric*—odd, aloof or suspicious. Includes paranoid and schizoid personality disorders.
• *Cluster B: dramatic* — emotionally labile, intense or erratic. Includes dissocial, emotionally unstable and histrionic personality disorders.
• *Cluster C: anxious* — constitutionally timid or worried. Includes avoidant, dependent and anankastic personality disorders.

The following vignettes illustrate the category and cluster approaches to personality disorder. They also highlight two important clinical points:
• Always describe clearly the characteristics upon which the diagnosis is being based.
• Always seek and record positive as well as negative attributes; the former are useful in management.

Miss D is 22 and has taken an impulsive overdose. She felt bored and angry with her boyfriend and various others. She has repeatedly self-harmed since early adolescence in response to minor life events — particularly when she feels abandoned. She reports having been sexually abused by her stepfather. Her lifestyle is chaotic and she misuses alcohol. Previous attempts to offer help have been thwarted by her failure to keep appointments. Her one enduring pleasure in life is looking after horses. Two days later she discharges herself; her boyfriend sent her some flowers and she is planning to marry him.

Table 15.1 ICD-10 personality disorders.

Paranoid — suspicion and distrust of others; sensitivity to criticism; stubbornness; self-importance
Schizoid — emotional detachment; introspection; social isolation; lack of humour
Dissocial (also called *psychopathic* or *antisocial*) — lack of concern for others; unstable relationships; low frustration threshold; irritability; aggression; failure to learn from experience; lack of guilt
Emotionally unstable (also called *borderline*) — multiple, turbulent relationships; impulsivity; repeated behavioural crises; variable mood; stress-related psychotic-like symptoms
Histrionic — exaggerated, theatrical expression of emotions; attention seeking; vain; crushes and fads
Anankastic (also called *obsessive–compulsive*) — excessive orderliness; preoccupation with detail; inflexible; dogmatic; humourless
Anxious (also called *avoidant*) — persistent feelings of tension and apprehension; avoidance of personal contact because of the fear of criticism or rejection
Dependent — a tendency to encourage others to make decisions; an excessive need to be taken care of
Organic — personality disorder after head injury (p. 135)
Three other categories, formerly included as personality disorders, are now considered to be variants of psychiatric disorders: *schizotypal* (p. 125), *depressive* (p. 87) and *cyclothymic* (p. 87)

Key features: impulsivity, sensitive to rejection, emotional instability.
Positive attributes: the care of animals. Has done unpaid work for an animal charity.
Cluster: dramatic.
ICD-10 category: emotionally unstable (borderline) personality disorder.

Dr E is a 60-year-old scientist who has accepted psychiatric referral under protest. He is unmarried and has had several brief, unsatisfactory relationships. He feels strongly that he has been denied the acclaim he deserves and is currently complaining bitterly to his head of department after unsuccessfully applying for promotion. He alleges that other workers steal his ideas. He does not mix with his colleagues and is uneasy in social gatherings.

Key features: socially isolated, suspicious, tendency to exaggerate self-importance.
Positive attributes: his research eminence shows a high level of functioning.
Cluster: eccentric.
ICD-10 category: paranoid personality disorder.

15.3 Management of personality disorders

15.3.1 General principles
Personality cannot be modified to any significant degree. Instead, management is aimed at tailoring the surroundings and circumstances to the personality.
• Reinforce skills and positive traits.
• Help the person find a lifestyle which suits them. For example, someone with anankastic personality disorder will do best in a job with a regular routine which requires steady, careful work.
• Avoid an inconsistent or excessive reaction to crises. Admissions are rarely helpful and may reinforce the behaviour. A consistent, limited and community-based approach is better.

• Many undesirable traits are exacerbated by substance misuse. Counselling and advice about this can help decrease acts of violence and self-harm.
• Treat any coexisting psychiatric disorder.

15.3.2 Management of eccentric (cluster A) personality disorder
Patients with 'eccentric'-type (cluster A) personality disorder are usually suspicious of mental health services and are unlikely to use them. Psychotherapy is ineffective and contraindicated.

15.3.3 Emotionally unstable (borderline) personality disorder
A patient like Miss D p. 147 may frequently attend her GP demanding benzodiazepines, take overdoses, misuse alcohol and have repeated brief admissions.
• Patients need a written care plan. Ensure good communication between the agencies involved to avoid 'splitting' (disagreements between staff induced by the patient — people with these personality traits induce a range of strong feelings). Respond to threats consistently and do not reinforce manipulative behaviour. Clear boundaries should be agreed about acceptable behaviour and about the nature of the service to be provided.
• An intensive form of psychotherapy (*dialectical behaviour therapy*) may be effective in reducing self-harm rates.
• SSRIs (or low-dose antipsychotics) can reduce impulsive behaviour, but their use is limited by the length of prescription likely to be necessary and the acceptability of medication.

15.3.4 Dissocial (psychopathic) disorder
• Historically, psychopathic disorder (as it is still called in legal circles) has had its own status: it is grounds for detention under the Mental Health Act (p. 73).
• In practice, psychiatrists rarely treat people with dissocial personality disorder (with or without consent) as no interventions have

been shown to be effective, and forensic problems are common.

• The main exception is that the Mental Health Act is used to send some people with dissocial personality disorder who have committed serious crimes to secure psychiatric hospitals rather than to prison. This is a controversial decision, affected by legal and social influences rather than by evidence of effectiveness. In hospital, prolonged psychotherapy or antipsychotic drugs may be tried.

15.3.5 Anxious (cluster C) personality disorder

There is little information about management of this cluster.

• Set realistic goals for treatment and avoid escalating contact which simply fosters dependency.

• Depressive disorder and neurosis are common. Both may precipitate a crisis and require treatment.

15.4 Epidemiology of personality disorders

The estimated prevalence of personality disorders in different settings is given in Table 15.2. These estimates are from studies using different methodologies and definitions and must be interpreted cautiously.

15.5 Aetiology of personality disorders

Very little is known of the aetiology of personality disorders, partly because so little is understood about the determinants of normal personality.

• There is a moderate genetic contribution to personality traits (e.g. 35–50% heritability for neuroticism and extraversion) and to some personality disorders, especially anankastic and dissocial types. Aggressive behaviour may be slightly commoner in men with sex chromosome abnormalities (especially XYY), but is much less so than sometimes portrayed.

• Upbringing and childhood experiences have major influences on our personality for better and worse. In particular, dissocial personality disorder is associated with adverse childhood events and poor parenting.

• Some patients with dissocial personality disorder have temporal lobe EEG abnormalities. *Minimal brain dysfunction* refers to the view that the disorder results from minor brain injury or delayed maturation.

15.6 Prognosis of personality disorders

The fact that personality disorders are considered to be lifelong and stable implies that prognosis is uniformly bad. In fact the

Table 15.2 The prevalence of personality disorders in different populations.

Setting	Type of personality disorder	Prevalence (%)
General population	All	13
	Dissocial (psychopathic)	4 (men); < 1 (women)
	Cluster A (eccentric)	1
	Cluster B (dramatic)	2–3
	Cluster C (anxious)	2–3
General practice	All	34
Psychiatric inpatients	All	49 (men); 40 (women)
	Emotionally unstable (borderline)	15

evidence suggests that considerable fluctuations do occur, and improvement is often observed by middle age. Some clinicians distinguish:
• *mature* personality disorders (corresponding to the eccentric cluster), which are first recognizable in late adolescence and which remain stable or worsen with age; from
• *immature* personality disorders (corresponding to the anxious and dramatic clusters), which have an onset in childhood and which mellow with age.

15.7 Personality disorder and psychiatric disorder

Personality and its disorders interact in important ways with psychiatric disorders:
• Personality disorder can *predispose to* psychiatric disorder. For example, people with anankastic personalities are vulnerable to depressive disorder.
• Personality disorder can *coexist with* psychiatric disorder (a type of comorbidity; p. 4) and worsens its prognosis.
• Personality disorder can be *mistaken for* psychiatric disorder (and vice versa). For example, someone with a depressive disorder may give the impression that they have a personality disorder (p. 14).
• Personality can be *affected by* psychiatric disorder. For example, in chronic schizophrenia (p. 115).
• Personality can have a *pathoplastic* effect on psychiatric disorder. That is, it can modify the clinical features even if it has no direct causal role. For example, obsessional personality traits are exaggerated in depressive disorder.

15.7.1 Multiaxial classification
These interactions have led some psychiatrists to advocate a *multiaxial* system in which psychiatric disorder and personality disorder are coded separately. Other axes record additional information.
Axis I — psychiatric disorder.

Axis II — personality disorder and mental retardation.
Axis III — general medical conditions.
Axis IV — psychosocial and environmental problems (i.e. the person's context).
Axis V — global assessment of functioning (rated on a 1–100 scale).

A 55-year-old man has lived alone in isolated and deprived surroundings all his life. He has developed delusions of persecution. He cannot read and has never worked. His mobility is limited. He improves moderately with treatment.

Axis I: delusional disorder.
Axis II: schizoid personality disorder; mild mental retardation.
Axis III: osteoarthritis.
Axis IV: homelessness, illiteracy.
Axis V: global assessment 25 (on admission); 45 (on discharge).
Multiaxial classification is part of DSM-IV. In the UK it is used mainly in child psychiatry (p. 152).

15.8 Problems with the concept of personality disorder

The very concept of personality disorder has been controversial because:
• It isn't a 'medical' category.
• It is unreliable.
• One person's personality disorder is another person's virtue. (Many famous people meet the criteria for personality disorder, yet the traits are either tolerated or are intrinsic to their success.)
• The term is pejorative — there is evidence that the label is applied to patients that doctors don't like or find hard to help.

Some of these issues clearly go beyond the boundaries of psychiatry. Given the current state of knowledge, psychiatrists must at least ensure that the term is used as reliably and usefully as possible.

15.9 SUMMARY: KEY POINTS

- Personality is the combination of emotional, cognitive and behavioural traits which characterize each of us. A personality is disordered if the traits cause problems for the individual or those around him.
- Personality disorders are classified pragmatically into three clusters: eccentric, anxious and dramatic.
- Emphasize positive attributes as well as negative ones.

- Personality disorder interacts with psychiatric disorder in five ways: as a predisposing factor; as a pathoplastic factor; as a prognostic factor; as a comorbid disorder; and as a differential diagnosis.
- Focus treatment on modifying circumstances, removing exacerbating factors and reinforcing positive behaviours.

CHAPTER 16

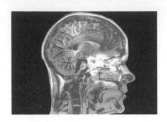

Childhood Disorders

16.1 Principles of child psychiatry

16.1.1 Interviewing children

When interviewing a child the objectives are the same as with adults: to establish rapport, to make a diagnosis, and to understand its aetiology and context. For several reasons, however, the nature of the interview differs:

• A child may not understand the question or may be unable to express himself.

• The range of disorders being sought, and hence the diagnostic focus, is different.

• Parents determine when and how the child presents.

• Family factors contribute to many disorders — so more attention is paid to the family.

Child psychiatry interviews have several features:

• Parents are present and often interviewed alone first to establish the history.

• The interviewer must be able to jump from one topic to another as led by the child.

• Assessment starts with play and non-threatening conversation to gain trust.

• Much information comes from the child's appearance and behaviour.

• Significant others (e.g. teachers, siblings) provide key parts of the history.

• Several sessions may be needed to complete the interview.

By adopting these strategies, the interviewer aims to collect information about all the topics in Table 16.1. In addition, a paediatric history and neurological examination may be indicated (e.g. if there is the possibility of a developmental disorder). To complete the assessment, background information is sought from relevant sources — teachers, siblings, social services.

• Get parental consent before carrying out an assessment or examination, unless abuse is suspected, in which case the duty of care to the child may override this principle (see p. 162).

• Consult a specialist text for further details about how to interview children.

16.1.2 Classification of child psychiatric disorders

The major psychiatric disorders of childhood are shown in Table 16.2.

A *multiaxial* scheme is often used to record the diagnostic information because of the importance of developmental stage, overall abilities and social circumstances:

Axis I — psychiatric disorder(s) present.

Axis II — developmental stage and delays.

Axis III — intellectual level.

Axis IV — medical problems.

Axis V — abnormal social situations.

• Mental retardation in children is covered in Chapter 17.

Presenting problem
    Onset, duration, factors affecting it
    Associated problems and symptoms
    Recent life events
    Parents' and child's explanation for it
Developmental milestones
    Motor — e.g. sitting, walking, toilet training
    Social — e.g. smiling
    Emotional — e.g. attachment behaviour
    Cognitive — e.g. talking, reading
    Other — e.g. toilet training
Emotional profile
    Temperament
    Problem behaviours
    Likes and dislikes
Family
    Relationship with parents and siblings
    Problems at home
    Separations from parents
Schooling
    Educational record
    Attendance
    Relationship with peers
General health
    Hospital admissions
    Previous psychiatric history
Observation of child
    General appearance
    Interactions with interviewer and family members present
    Attention and concentration
    Prevailing mood and range of emotions expressed
    Language and motor skills

Table 16.1 Topics for the child psychiatric interview.

Table 16.2 Childhood psychiatric disorders.

Emotional disorders (neuroses)
    Anxiety disorders
    Somatoform disorder
Behavioural disorders
    Conduct disorder
    Hyperkinetic disorder
Depressive disorder
Developmental disorders
    Autism
    Specific reading disorder
Miscellaneous conditions
    Enuresis
    Encopresis
    Elective mutism
    Tics

16.1.3 Epidemiology of child psychiatric disorder

Transient symptoms and behavioural disturbances are common in children of all ages. The major epidemiological features of childhood psychiatric disorder are:

• Prevalence at age 10 is 7% in rural areas, 13% in urban areas. At age 14 the prevalence is higher.

• Boys are affected twice as often as girls for most diagnoses.

• Commonest diagnoses are emotional and conduct disorder.

• Disorders are commoner in children with mental retardation, epilepsy or medical illnesses.

16.1.4 Aetiology in child psychiatry

The same broad range of aetiological factors operate in childhood as in adulthood (Chapter 6; Table 16.3).

- There is a genetic component to most disorders, mediated partly through its influence on temperament and intelligence.
- The major environmental factors are the family and social circumstances.

16.1.5 Management in child psychiatry

Management of children with psychiatric disorder is based upon several principles:

- Take the child's developmental stage and overall level of functioning into account.
- Most problems are treated initially with reassurance, support and behavioural interventions.
- Whatever the treatment, involve the family.
- Avoid removal from school or home wherever possible.
- Medication has a limited role in most disorders.

Further details are discussed in the sections describing the specific disorders.

- The organization of child psychiatric services was mentioned on p. 78.

Table 16.3 Causative factors in child psychiatry.

Factor	Examples
Genetic	Autism
Environmental	
Family factors	
Parenting styles	Harsh, critical style associated with conduct disorder
Parental conflict or separation	Increased risk of emotional or conduct disorder
Parental psychiatric disorder	
Social factors	
Deprivation	
Other factors	
Medical disorder	Epilepsy increases risk of most disorders
Physical abuse	

Table 16.4 Prognosis of psychiatric disorders in childhood.

Category	Long-term outcome
Emotional disorders	Good. Two-thirds resolve in a 4-year period
Mood disorder	Poor. Half have depressive disorder in adulthood
Behavioural disorders	
Conduct disorder	Poor. Often leads to personality disorder or substance abuse
Hyperkinetic disorder	Variable
Developmental disorders	
Autism	Lifelong
Specific reading disorder	Moderate
Other conditions	
Enuresis	Good
Encopresis	Good
Tics	Usually transient (unless Tourette syndrome)
Elective mutism	Uncertain

16.1.6 Prognosis in child psychiatry

Childhood psychiatric disorders have a variable outcome, in part because of the influence of the child's ongoing development and experiences. The overall pattern is summarized in Table 16.4.

16.2 Emotional disorders

Neuroses (emotional disorders) were described in Chapter 10. In children, the disorders are in many ways similar, and most of the individual subtypes are recognized. However, there are important differences between the disorders in children and in adults:
• 'Emotional disorder' rather than 'neurosis' is the usual term.
• Some subtypes are different (e.g. separation anxiety).
• Medication is rarely used.
• Equal male : female ratio (cf. 1 : 2 in adults).
• Most affected children do not become affected adults.

16.2.1 Anxiety disorders

Crying when mummy leaves the room, or becoming fearful of animals, are anxieties which children normally experience at particular developmental stages, especially at times of stress and transition. They must be distinguished from persistent, significant symptoms warranting a diagnosis of anxiety disorder. The latter affect 5% of children at some time. As in adults, anxiety manifests itself as behavioural, psychological and physical symptoms (Table 16.5).

Separation anxiety

Among 5–11-year-olds 3–4% have excessive, prolonged anxiety when faced with separation from parents or others they are attached to. The child clings — literally or metaphorically — to the person and tries to avoid being separated from them. Sleep disturbance and nightmares occur. Older children may describe being fearful that the person will be harmed and will not return. Separation anxiety often

Table 16.5 Symptoms of anxiety in children.

Behavioural
    Clinging to parent
    Unwilling to leave house
    Unwilling to go to bed
    Actions designed to avoid feared event (e.g. hiding)
Psychological
    Feeling worried
    Nightmares
Physical
    Abdominal pain
    Headaches

begins at times of stress, such as after the death of the family dog. Some parents are noted to be overprotective. Management includes:
• Explanation and reassurance.
• Identification and resolution of stressors.
• Ensuring the parents are not reinforcing the problem (e.g. by appearing anxious when about to leave the child).
• Use of specific interventions for secondary problems such as school refusal which may develop.
• Applying behavioural techniques (p. 67) such as gradually increasing the time and distance between parent and child.

16.2.2 Somatoform disorder

Children readily develop somatic symptoms, especially when stressed. Non-specific abdominal pain and headaches are the commonest and may lead initially to a paediatric referral. As in adults, *somatoform disorder* describes persistent unexplained bodily symptoms (p. 102). The assessment centres upon:
• Exclusion of an underlying emotional or depressive disorder.
• Identification of precipitating and perpetuating factors. For example, the child may be unhappy at home, worried about a sick sibling, or using the symptoms to gain attention.

Management is aimed at avoiding reinforcing the symptoms and at tackling the underlying stresses. The prognosis is variable — some patients go on to have somatoform disorders as adults.

16.2.3 Other emotional disorders

Obsessive–compulsive disorder in children is rare but serious. It may be associated with Tourette syndrome (p. 160).

• It is the only childhood emotional disorder for which there is good evidence that medication (clomipramine, fluoxetine) and psychological (cognitive behavioural) therapy are effective. Nevertheless, the prognosis in severe cases is quite poor.

Children also suffer from the other emotional disorders seen in adults (Chapter 10). For example, they can get *specific phobias* or develop emotional disorders following particular stresses (*adjustment reactions*).

• The occurrence and management of *chronic fatigue syndrome* in children is currently under debate.

16.2.4 School refusal

Many children try to avoid going to school from time to time. Some do it regularly. School refusal is not a psychiatric disorder, but it is a common cause of referral to a child psychiatrist and is frequently attributable to an emotional disorder. Its assessment is summarized in Table 16.6.

First, exclude truancy and parental behaviour as causes for the absence from school. The characteristics of school refusal and truancy are different (Table 16.7). School refusal is usually a manifestation of separation anxiety, often provoked by recent events at home or at school. In older children, school refusal may reflect bullying; it can also herald a more pervasive problem such as social phobia or depressive disorder.

Management is aimed at a rapid return to school before avoidance is too ingrained. Sometimes a graded re-exposure is needed. Address any specific fears or stresses, and treat any associated psychiatric disorder.

The prognosis in younger children is good. In older children, the problem may become prolonged and other psychiatric problems may emerge. There is a slightly increased risk of anxiety disorder in adulthood.

Table 16.6 Assessment of suspected school refusal.

Why is the child absent from school?
School refusal
Truancy
Parents keeping child at home
Physical illness

What does the school refusal reflect?
Reluctance to leave home (i.e. secondary to separation anxiety)
A specific 'school phobia' (e.g. of getting there or of being bullied)
A more generalized disorder (e.g. social phobia, depressive disorder)

What are the other factors affecting the presentation or management?
Recent life events (e.g. bereavement)
Recent events at school (e.g. change of class)
Parental characteristics (e.g. overprotective)

16.3 Mood disorders

The occurrence of mood disorder in children has been a controversial area. It is now thought

Table 16.7 Distinguishing school refusal from truancy.

School refusal	Truancy
Younger (< 11 years old)	Older (> 11 years old)
Underlying emotional disorder	Underlying conduct disorder
Good academic and behavioural record	Poor school record
Good prognosis	Poor prognosis
Parents overprotective and anxious	Broken home

that depressive disorders, but not bipolar disorder, exist in prepubertal and even preschool children. The prevalence prior to adolescence is low, estimated at < 1%. Similar principles apply when making the diagnosis of depression in a child as in an adult:

• Symptoms present for at least 2 weeks.
• If there are also symptoms of emotional disorder, attempt to distinguish the primary diagnosis.
• Depressive disorders are classified using the adult system (p. 83).

The aetiology of childhood depressive disorder involves the same mixture of genes, life events and unknown influences as prevail in adult cases.

Management includes support, monitoring and reducing stressors. Neither antidepressants nor psychological treatments have been shown unequivocally to be effective, but both are used. The prognosis is poor; in many the condition becomes chronic and half suffer from depressive disorder in adulthood.

In *adolescents*, depressive disorder has a prevalence of 3–4%. Cognitive behavioural therapy is the treatment of choice. Antidepressants are widely prescribed with best evidence for fluoxetine. The risk of suicide becomes significant and admission may be necessary. ECT is used rarely and controversially.

Conduct is disturbed and antisocial, well beyond the range of misbehaviour normally observed (Table 16.8). Diagnosis is usually made after the age of 7, though problems have often been apparent before the age of 5. The term *oppositional defiant disorder* is used for these younger children.

• A distinction is sometimes made between *socialized conduct disorder*, where the activities occur within a peer group, and *unsocialized conduct disorder*, where the child acts in isolation.

In adolescence, conduct disorder has a strong relationship with juvenile delinquency and substance misuse. There is often repeated police contact and convictions for theft, criminal damage or assault.

Conduct disorder is associated with a variety of indices of social deprivation and poor parenting (Table 16.9). Any genetic contribution is small.

The long-term prognosis is poor; 50% of cases progress to dissocial personality disorder (p. 147), and persistent substance misuse and criminality are common. Those who form stable relationships have a better outcome.

There is no specific management and no convincing evidence that any intervention affects outcome. In practice, management is a mixture of attempts to treat and to punish:

16.4 Behavioural disorders

Behavioural disorders are diagnosed in children who are persistently and excessively naughty. The major distinction is between behavioural problems which result from overactivity (hyperkinetic disorder) and those which do not (conduct disorder). Neither label should be applied unless the diagnostic criteria are met — all children are naughty and 'hyper' from time to time.

16.4.1 Conduct disorder

Conduct disorder is the commonest psychiatric disorder of childhood and adolescence. It occurs mainly in boys (sex ratio 5 : 1).

Table 16.8 Clinical features of conduct disorder.

In preschool children
Aggressive behaviour
Poor concentration
In mid-childhood
Lying
Stealing
Disruptive and oppositional behaviour
Bullying
In adolescence
Stealing
Truancy
Promiscuity
Substance misuse
Vandalism
Reckless behaviour

Table 16.9 Factors associated with conduct disorder.

Family factors
Parental personality disorder
Parental alcoholism
Parental disputes and violence
Harsh, inconsistent parenting
Being in care early in life
Large family size
Social factors
Inner cities
Deprivation and overcrowding
Individual factors
Brain damage
Epilepsy
Specific reading disorder

Table 16.10 Features of hyperkinetic disorder.

Core features
Hyperactive
Poor attention and concentration
Distractible
Impulsive
Poor at planning and organizing tasks
Onset by age 9, usually by 5
Associated features
Learning difficulties
Clumsiness
Low self-esteem
Socially disinhibited
Unpopular with other children
Non-localizing neurological signs
Conduct disorder coexists in 50%

- Family therapy seeks to improve the home environment, and includes teaching parents how to cope with the behaviour and reduce conflict. The child may be offered one-to-one sessions when causes for the behaviour are discussed and strategies for controlling it are taught.
- Alternative outlets for energies and behaviours are sought (e.g. youth clubs, car workshops).
- Problems such as truancy and substance misuse should be dealt with appropriately, preferably before they become established.
- Residential care is occasionally used.

16.4.2 Hyperkinetic disorder

Also called *attention deficit hyperactivity disorder*. The clinical features are shown in Table 16.10. As with conduct disorder, the diagnosis requires that the problem is both persistent and extreme. In UK the prevalence is 2%; three-quarters are boys.
- In the USA, where less stringent criteria are used, prevalence and treatment rates are correspondingly higher.

The aetiology of hyperkinetic disorder is multifactorial:
- There is a modest genetic contribution. Families also show increased rates of depressive disorder, learning difficulties, alcoholism and antisocial personality disorder.

- A neurodevelopmental abnormality is suspected, on the basis of the neurological signs and learning difficulties, and from brain imaging and EEG findings.
- There is an association with social deprivation, though less striking than for conduct disorder.
- Many parents blame food allergy, but this is rarely demonstrable when investigated properly.

The management of hyperkinetic disorder involves:
- Support for the child and family.
- Specific educational approaches, including attention to associated learning difficulties.
- Firm adherence to behavioural principles (to reward good behaviour and discourage hyperactive behaviour).
- Stimulants, usually *methylphenidate*, which have an important role. This paradoxical but effective treatment originated from the (incorrect) belief that the disorder reflects a failure of cortical arousal. Side-effects are insomnia, poor appetite and headaches. Use has been limited in the UK by concerns about addiction and growth retardation but is becoming more widespread.

Prognosis is variable. Gradual improvement occurs in adolescence and a third of cases resolve entirely. The rest have residual hyperkinetic features, especially those with learning difficulties or conduct disorder. Development of dissocial personality disorder and substance misuse are common.

16.5 Developmental disorders

Developmental disorders can be *pervasive* or *specific*. The former affect many aspects of psychological and neurobiological development; *autism* is the commonest type. In specific developmental disorder, there is impairment in only one domain (e.g. reading) relative to overall development. These seemingly diverse conditions are grouped together for three reasons:
• their onset is always during infancy or early childhood;
• the abnormality is thought to be directly related to brain development; and
• their course lacks the fluctuations of most psychiatric disorders.

16.5.1 Pervasive developmental disorders — autism

Autism is characterized by a failure to develop normal communication, especially social and emotional communication. Autistic children have a delayed and restricted use of language, and seem oblivious to non-verbal cues and emotional expressions. They have no desire to interact with others or form relationships. Instead, they demonstrate a limited range of solitary, repetitive behaviours and resist attempts to change their routine. The features are summarized in Table 16.11.

Table 16.11 Features of autism.

1 in 2500 children; 80% boys.
Age of onset <3 years
Key clinical features (the '*autistic triad*')
No emotional warmth (autistic aloneness)
Impaired language and communication
Solitary, repetitive behaviours
Associated features
Mannerisms and rituals
Epilepsy in 25%
Mental retardation in 75%
Non-specific behavioural problems

• A few autistic children, called *idiots savants*, have remarkable abilities in discrete areas, such as complex mental arithmetic (as in the film *Rain Man*).

The differential diagnosis is from other pervasive developmental disorders with autistic features such as *Asperger's syndrome*, *Rett's syndrome* (which affects girls) and *disintegrative psychosis*. Also consider separate causes of a failure to develop communication, such as specific language disorder, mental retardation or deafness.

The aetiology of autism is strongly genetic. The causative genes have not been identified. No environmental risk factors are known (cf. p. 52). Neuropathological involvement of the cerebellum and olivary nuclei has been reported.

The prognosis is poor. Speech eventually develops in some, but communication remains limited and the core abnormalities rarely improve. Seizures can occur later in childhood. Most autistic children need special schooling and residential care, and only a minority are ever able to live independently.

There is no specific treatment. The main components of management are:
• making the diagnosis;
• supporting the family;
• providing appropriate accommodation and education; and
• dealing with abnormal behaviours.

16.5.2 Specific developmental disorders

Specific developmental disorders are conditions in which there is marked delay in one area of development relative to the child's overall IQ — usually reading, also arithmetic, language or motor skills. Though the 'symptoms' are not really psychiatric, children may be referred to child psychiatric services because of associated emotional or behavioural problems.

Specific reading disorder
In specific reading disorder, reading skills are significantly (> 2 standard deviations) below that predicted by the child's overall

performance. Visual impairment or lack of education must be excluded as the cause. It affects 4% of 10-year-olds, and is four times commoner in boys than girls.

• It is associated with conduct disorder in a third of cases, and with low social class and a disturbed family background. The direction of causality between these factors is unclear.

• Assessment is by an educational psychologist using standardized tests (though this service is not always available).

• Management involves restoration of morale and reward-driven remedial teaching.

• Prognosis is poor, with reading abilities often remaining well below average.

16.6 Other conditions

16.6.1 Enuresis

Enuresis is urinary incontinence after the age at which bladder control is expected (*primary enuresis*; must be at least 5 years old) or where there has previously been normal continence (*secondary enuresis*). It usually presents as bed-wetting in the first half of the night (*nocturnal enuresis*). It affects 10% of 5-year-olds, 2% of 10-year-olds and 1% of 14-year-olds. Boys out-number girls 3 : 1.

• Enuresis can cause great distress, interfere with normal activities (e.g. staying at a friend's house) and lead to the child being bullied.

In the assessment, exclude (and treat) urinary tract infection, diabetes or neurological disorder. Search for recent stressors and symptoms of emotional disorder (twice as common as expected in those with enuresis). There is often a history of enuresis in male relatives.

Management includes:

• Reassurance and explanation (to child and parent).

• Treatment of associated psychiatric disorder.

• Behavioural methods. A *star chart* is the best treatment for younger children: they are rewarded for dryness with stars or another suitable token. (A good example of operant conditioning; p. 53.) An *enuresis alarm* ('pad and buzzer') is a moisture-sensitive pad worn by the child. When urine is passed, a buzzer goes off which wakes the child in time to go to the toilet to finish. He also participates in changing the sheets. An alarm is usually effective if persisted with for several weeks, especially in children over 6 years old.

• Pharmacological methods. Tricyclic antidepressants (e.g. imipramine 25–50 mg nocte) work, but relapse is common. Intranasal desmopressin has similar efficacy and fewer side-effects.

The prognosis is good though a few boys remain enuretic into adulthood.

16.6.2 Encopresis

Encopresis is the passing of faeces in an inappropriate place after age 4. As with enuresis it can be *primary* or *secondary*. Children may soil their pants, pass faeces in hidden places or occasionally smear them.

At assessment, exclude problems due to diarrhoea, constipation, Hirschsprung's disease, other physical cause and mental retardation.

• There is often a history of inadequate or harsh toilet training combined with recent stresses and emotional disorder in the child.

Management is by reassurance, help with associated problems and ensuring that the parents do not become punitive. The standard behavioural manoeuvre is to toilet the child after each meal, and reward him for staying there, for producing a motion and for not soiling. Encopresis rarely occurs beyond mid-teens.

16.6.3 Tics

Tics are involuntary, rapid, spasmodic movements, usually repeated blinking and grimacing. They are common, especially in young boys, and may begin after an emotional upset. They are generally transient and need no specific treatment. However, some tics become severe, prolonged and incapacitating.

The main tic disorder is (*Gilles de la*) *Tourette syndrome*, in which tics are accompanied by vocal grunts and expletives (*coprolalia*). Obses-

sive–compulsive symptoms often occur. Boys are affected more than girls (3 : 1). Incidence is 1/2000. Drug treatment is with low-dose antipsychotics. Though the tics usually diminish in adulthood, the other symptoms may persist.
• Tourette's syndrome has a genetic basis which overlaps with that of obsessive–compulsive disorder.

16.6.4 Elective mutism
In elective mutism, also called *selective mutism*, children refuse to speak although able to do so. Speech is usually normal at home but absent elsewhere. Non-verbal communication is preserved. Onset is from 4 to 8 years of age. Affected children tend to be shy, anxious and isolated in most settings, but aggressive and behaviourally disturbed at home. The disorder is rare, and is unusual in that it is commoner in girls than boys. It is said to be associated with overprotective parents and depressed mothers.
• There is no specific treatment; a range of behavioural interventions may be tried.
• Elective mutism can persist for several years, but the long-term prognosis is unknown.

16.6.5 Psychoses in childhood and adolescence
Schizophrenia may begin in adolescence, and occasionally in younger children. *Bipolar disorder* can also start in adolescence.
• These disorders are treated in a similar fashion to adult-onset cases (and are one of the few clear indications for medication in child psychiatry).

16.7 Special groups

16.7.1 Toddlers
Toddlers are rightly notorious for *temper tantrums*. Reassurance that this is normal and simple advice on limit setting are usually all that is needed. Consistency in the parents' response to the behaviour is crucial. Self-help books are available.
Sleep disturbances are common, either

refusal to settle, or night-time waking due to *night terrors* and *nightmares*. Use reassurance and a consistent bedtime routine. Psychiatric referral is rare, though occasionally the disturbances herald an emotional or behavioural disorder.

16.7.2 Teenagers
Contrary to the stereotype, neither emotional turmoil nor delinquency are normal for teenagers. Persistently withdrawn, disruptive or bizarre behaviour should be assessed to exclude psychiatric disorder. Diagnostically, adolescents get the tail end of childhood disorders, and the early onset of adult disorders (Table 16.12), so the clinician must be knowledgeable about both and the continuities between them. This has led to the delineation of *adolescent psychiatry* as a subspecialty.

Table 16.12 Important psychiatric disorders of adolescence.

Conduct disorder
Eating disorder
Substance misuse disorders (especially alcohol, ecstasy, glue)
Depressive disorder
Anxiety disorder
Schizophrenia
Bipolar disorder
Deliberate self-harm

16.7.3 Children in care
Children in care, especially in children's homes, have high rates of psychiatric disorder, notably conduct disorder, substance misuse and self-harm. This may be both a cause and a consequence of being in care.

16.7.4 Children with physical illness
Children with chronic medical illness are at increased risk of psychiatric disorder. This is especially true for organic brain syndromes and epilepsy. The associations may reflect partly a common aetiology, but also the effects of physical illness on the child's intellectual, psychological and social development.

• Close co-operation between those involved in the psychiatric and medical disorders is essential.

16.7.5 Children with psychiatrically ill parents

If a parent has a psychiatric disorder, the child is at risk of psychiatric problems via an increased likelihood of inadequate or abnormal parenting, as well as from inheritance of a genetic predisposition. Hence the mental health (and personality) of parents is part of the child psychiatric assessment (Table 16.1). Specific parental problems associated with particular outcomes in the child include:

• maternal substance misuse affecting fetal development;
• paternal alcoholism and conduct disorder;
• maternal depression impairing child's development;
• maternal eating disorder and abnormal feeding of child; and
• Munchausen's syndrome by proxy — parent fabricating symptoms or signs in the child.

16.7.6 Abused children

Children can be abused sexually, physically or emotionally. The abuse has psychiatric as well as medical and legal repercussions. Key points concerning the psychiatric aspects of child abuse are:

• Take specialist advice whenever abuse is suspected. This may be obtained from paediatricians, child psychiatrists and social services' child protection teams.

• Children who are being abused may show physical, psychological or behavioural stigmata.
• Managing abused children is difficult and needs multidisciplinary input. Child psychiatrists have particular roles in identifying and treating the psychological consequences of the abuse. It is unknown whether intervention alters the long-term prognosis for the abused (or the abuser).
• *Physical abuse* (*non-accidental injury*) causes significant morbidity and mortality. Either the child or the abuser may need to be removed from the home. Physical abuse leads to higher rates of emotional and behavioural disorder.
• Children who are *emotionally abused* (neglected) have delayed psychological and physical development and increased rates of emotional disturbance. In extreme cases, they may present with failure to thrive (*deprivation dwarfism*).

The effects of abuse may continue into adulthood:

• Women who were sexually abused have double the risk of psychiatric disorder and five-fold higher rates of psychiatric admission. Borderline personality disorder (p. 147) and possibly bulimia nervosa appear to be particularly common. There are no good data on the outcome for sexually abused boys — apart from their risk of becoming abusers and perpetuating the cycle.
• Emotional abuse may lead to persistent low self-esteem, relationship difficulties and personality disorder.

16.8 SUMMARY: KEY POINTS

• Conduct disorder and emotional disorder are the commonest psychiatric diagnoses in children. The former tends to do badly, the latter well.
• When making a diagnosis, take both the child's development stage and the parents' role into account.

• The risk of child psychiatric disorder is greater in urban areas, in boys, and in children with mental retardation or chronic illnesses.
• Treatment is usually behavioural and is aimed at the family as well as at the child.

CHAPTER 17

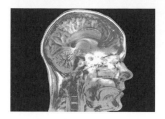

Mental Retardation
(Learning Disability)

17.1 Principles

17.1.1 Definition and key features

Mental retardation, mental handicap, mental subnormality, developmental disability and *learning disability* are synonyms. Mental retardation is the ICD-10 term, though learning disability is often preferred.

Mental retardation is defined as:

- IQ below 70;
- impairment across a wide range of functions; and
- onset in childhood.

The features of mental retardation are shown in Table 17.1. It must be distinguished from:

- lower than average intelligence but IQ greater than 70;
- specific developmental disorders (p. 159); and
- intellectual impairment secondary to an adult organic syndrome (p. 135).

The incidence of mental retardation has declined because of medical advances (e.g. immunization) and termination of affected pregnancies; the prevalence has not changed because of improved survival rates.

Mild mental retardation represents the tail end of the normal population distribution for intelligence and, as such, results from an interaction between multiple genetic and environmental factors. A specific cause is more often identifiable in severe cases.

17.1.2 Clinical features of mental retardation

Mental retardation can be *mild, moderate* or *severe* (Table 17.2). Its cause, if known, is coded separately.

A *profound* category (IQ < 20) is sometimes used as well.

17.1.3 Assessment of mental retardation

The presence of mental retardation may be suspected:

- before birth — due to pregnancy complications or results of antenatal tests;
- at birth — from the physical appearance; or
- after birth — from delayed milestones.

Assessment of a child with suspected mental retardation encompasses:

- making the diagnosis — establishing its presence, severity and likely cause (similar to the steps in evaluation of dementia; and
- evaluating concurrent psychiatric problems.

The areas of assessment are listed in Table 17.3. Practicalities depend on the child's age and the circumstances of the assessment. There is a special emphasis on the obstetric and neurodevelopmental history and on the physical examination.

- Diagnosis of the cause of the mental retardation involves paediatricians and paediatric neurologists.

163

Divided into mild, moderate, severe and profound forms
Prevalence is about 2%, with a male : female ratio of 3 : 2
Usually untreatable
Often accompanied by:
  psychiatric disorder
  behavioural disturbance
  medical problems (e.g. epilepsy)
Causes:
  a variety of genetic and environmental factors commonest
  specific causes are Down's syndrome and fragile X syndrome

Table 17.1 Features of mental retardation.

Table 17.2 Features of mild, moderate and severe mental retardation.

	Mild	Moderate	Severe
IQ range	69–50	49–35	< 35
Percentage of cases	85%	10%	5%
Ability to self-care	Independent	Need some help	Limited
Language	Reasonable	Limited	Basic or none
Reading and writing	Reasonable	Basic	Minimal or none
Ability to work	Semi-skilled	Unskilled, supervised	Supervised basic tasks
Social skills	Normal	Moderate	Few
Physical problems	Rare	Sometimes	Common
Aetiology discovered	Sometimes	Often	Usually

17.1.4 Psychiatric aspects of mental retardation

Children and adults with mental retardation have high rates (about 40%) of behavioural disturbance and psychiatric disorder. The risk is increased to 60% by coexistent epilepsy, and decreased in Down's syndrome.

Psychiatric disorder in mentally retarded children

All the main psychiatric disorders are commoner in mentally retarded children. Assessment is based on the principles of the child psychiatric assessment (p. 153) modified according to intellectual level (Table 17.4).

Psychiatric disorder in mentally retarded adults

An adult with mental retardation may require psychiatric assessment for a number of reasons:

• To assess the level of functioning and nature of current problems in order to help plan future management (e.g. placement).

• To assess and characterize a behavioural problem — called a *challenging behaviour* — such as shouting or inappropriate sexual activities.

• To investigate a suspected psychiatric disorder, such as schizophrenia or depression. These occur more commonly than in the general population, and their recognition is difficult because of the mental retardation; various scales have been devised to help. Trials of medication may be needed.

• As part of a forensic or risk assessment. People with mental retardation sometimes commit arson or other dangerous acts.

• To assess a decline in abilities. This may reflect the progressive nature of the condition or a superimposed disorder (e.g. depression).

Table 17.3 Assessment of mental retardation.

History
Details of pregnancy
Fetal growth
Infections, trauma, eclampsia
Substance misuse
Delivery
Gestational age
Complications
Condition of baby
Child's development
Milestones
Physical difficulties
Family history
Mental retardation
Physical anomalies
Consanguinity of parents
Examination
General
Overall health
Weight, height, head circumference
Physical anomalies and stigmata
Neurological
Tone, posture, power, reflexes
Cranial nerves
Motor skills
Comprehension and use of language
Neuropsychological testing
Intelligence quotient (IQ)
Language development
Laboratory investigations
Karyotyping and genetic testing
Biochemical studies
Brain imaging
(Prenatal screening: amniocentesis, chorionic
villus sampling)

Table 17.4 Psychiatric assessment in mental retardation.

Background
Overall level of functioning
Associated physical handicaps
Cause of mental retardation
Psychiatric history
Normal temperament and behaviours
Recent changes in environment
Recent changes in behaviour
Examination
Interactions
Attention
Perseverance
Mood
Presence and nature of emotional
expression
Features of autism
Investigations
Behavioural rating scales
Autistic rating scales

- prevailing temperament and behaviour; and
- level of support from family.

Management of learning disability uses the approaches employed elsewhere in psychiatry:

- Most patients are now looked after in the community. 'Normalization' is a phrase often used. Residential care is reserved for the most severely affected.
- Care is provided by multidisciplinary community learning disability teams using a framework similar to community mental health teams p. 76. Voluntary agencies play an important role.
- Services for dealing with challenging behaviours are organized at local and regional levels.

17.1.5 Management

Half of those with mental retardation do not require any specific service provision, mostly because they are at the mild end of the spectrum. Amongst the rest, there is a vast difference in the nature and amount of support needed, a variability determined by:

- overall level of functioning;
- ability in specific domains (e.g. language, toileting, cooking);
- physical handicaps;
- coexisting psychiatric disorder;

17.2 Conditions associated with mental retardation

The main individual causes of mental retardation are mentioned here. By and large, aetiology does not markedly affect management, but it may have major implications for the prognosis and the likelihood of similar problems arising in other family members.

17.2.1 Chromosomal abnormalities
Down's syndrome

Down's syndrome (trisomy 21) involves mental retardation and characteristic physical features (Table 17.5). The diagnosis is usually made at or before birth.

Down's syndrome is the commonest cause of mental retardation. Its incidence is 1 in 650 live births, the risk rising from < 1 in 2000 at maternal age 20 to 1 in 30 at age 45.

The aetiology in 95% of cases is triplication of chromosome 21, with the syndrome presumed to result from expression of the extra copy of the genes on the chromosome. The remaining cases are due to a translocation involving chromosome 21 or to mosaicism (a mixture of normal and trisomic cells).

The prognosis has improved with better medical management. Many people survive to middle age, when intellectual decline due to Alzheimer's disease is common. The association between the two disorders was crucial in the discovery of the latter's genetic basis (p. 127).

Fragile X syndrome

Fragile X syndrome is so called because of a fragile site on the long arm of the X chromosome seen when cells are grown in a folate-deficient medium. It occurs in about 1/1500 births and is the second commonest cause of mental retardation (~ 10% of cases). Its exact prevalence is uncertain because its phenotype (Table 17.6) is variable and accurate genetic testing has only recently become possible.

Most cases of fragile X syndrome are due to a triplet repeat mutation in the FMR1 gene. As this is on the X chromosome the syndrome is commoner in boys than girls (explaining much of the excess mental retardation in males). However, the unusual nature of the mutation means that some males who have the mutation are normal, and more females are affected than would be expected. Female carriers also have an increased risk of psychiatric disorders. The disorder gets worse in succeeding generations (*anticipation*).
- Genetic detection of affected individuals and carriers is now feasible.
- There is no specific treatment. *Methylphenidate* and *folic acid* may improve the attentional deficits.

Table 17.5 Features of Down's syndrome.

Moderate or severe mental retardation
Placid temperament
Physical features
Slanted eyes and epicanthic folds
Small mouth with furrowed tongue
Flat nose
Flattened occiput
Stubby hands with single transverse palmar crease
Hypotonia
Associated medical problems
Cardiac septal defects
Gastrointestinal obstruction
Atlantoaxial instability
Susceptibility to infection
Increased incidence of lymphoma and hypothyroidism

Table 17.6 Features of fragile X syndrome.

Commoner in males (> 2 : 1)
All features are particularly variable
Mental retardation
May be mild, moderate, severe or profound
Gets worse late in childhood
Performance IQ affected more than verbal IQ
'Litany speech' — repetitive; lacking in themes or content
Poor attention and concentration
Autistic features common
Physical features
Large, protruding ears
Long face with high-arched palate
Flat feet
Lax joints
Soft skin
Large testes (after puberty)
Mitral valve prolapse

Other chromosomal abnormalities

Severe mental retardation is common in other abnormalities of the autosomal chromosomes, but less frequent in abnormalities of the sex chromosomes.

• *Prader–Willi syndrome* is mental retardation together with compulsive eating, obesity, disruptive behaviour and hypogonadism. It is due to deletion of part of chromosome 15. *Angelman's syndrome* (severe retardation, puppet-like movements, laughter and a big tongue), is caused by the same abnormality when inherited from mother rather than father.

17.2.2 Single gene disorders

Phenylketonuria

Phenylketonuria (PKU) is the classic inborn error of metabolism (Table 17.7). The amino acid phenylalanine cannot be converted into paratyrosine because of a defective converting enzyme. It is autosomal recessive and affects 1/10 000 live births, causing 1% of severe mental retardation.

Table 17.7 Features of phenylketonuria.

Severe mental retardation
Tantrums and unpredictable aggression
Abnormal movements and mannerisms
Fair skin
Short stature
Associated medical problems
Eczema
Vomiting
Seizures

Table 17.8 Examples of metabolic disorders associated with mental retardation.

Metabolic category	Example
Amino acids	Homocysteinuria
Lipids	Tay–Sachs disease
Mucopolysaccharides	Hurler's syndrome
Carbohydrates	Galactosaemia
Purines	Lesch–Nyhan syndrome

Table 17.9 Pre- and perinatal environmental causes of mental retardation.

Category	Comment
Obstetric complications	
In utero infections	
Rubella	Greatest risk (50%) if infection is in first trimester
HIV	Retardation in 50% of infected children. Most die in a few years
Syphilis	
Cytomegalovirus	
Toxoplasmosis	
Fetal alcohol syndrome	In some offspring of mothers who drink heavily
Placental insufficiency	
Placental abruption	
Eclampsia/toxaemia	
Birth complications	May be a consequence of earlier fetal abnormality
Ventricular haemorrhage	
Perinatal factors	
Hypothyroidism (cretinism)	An important cause in areas with low iodine diets
Hyperbilirubinaemia	
Other factors	
Cerebral palsy	
Hydrocephalus	Mental retardation commoner than expected, though many individuals have normal IQ
Spina bifida	

• PKU is one of the few treatable causes of mental retardation, if a rigorous low phenylalanine diet is started in the first months of life—hence the neonatal screening for phenylalanine levels. Carriers can be detected.

Other inherited errors of metabolism

Mental retardation can result from disorders of other metabolic pathways (Table 17.8). The frequency of each condition is low and varies between ethnic groups. Most are associated with failure to thrive and hepatic and/or renal dysfunction. In *Lesch–Nyhan syndrome*, self-mutilation by biting is characteristic.

• All the cited examples are autosomal recessive and most can be detected prenatally. A few can be ameliorated by diet.

Other genetic disorders

Neurofibromatosis and *tuberous sclerosis complex* are neurocutaneous syndromes. Both are autosomal dominant but spontaneous mutations are common.

• *Neurofibromatosis* (von Recklinghausen's disease) affects 1/5000 births. Diagnostic features are *café au lait* spots on the skin and multiple neurofibromas. Mild mental retardation can occur in type I neurofibromatosis, which is due to a mutation in the NFI gene on chromosome 17.

• *Tuberous sclerosis complex* (TSC) occurs in 1/6000 births. There are several characteristic skin lesions and multiple tumours in brain and elsewhere. Epilepsy and progressive mental retardation occur in 60%. Autistic features are often seen. TSC genes are on chromosomes 9 and 16.

17.2.3 Environmental factors

Mental retardation is associated with a variety of environmental insults. Most act pre- or perinatally (Table 17.9) but postnatal factors are also recognized (Table 17.10).

Table 17.10 Postnatal causes of mental retardation.

Infections
Meningitis
Encephalitis
Brain tumours
Head injury
Accidental
Non-accidental
Hypoxia (e.g. anaesthetic accident)
Lead poisoning
Rare idiopathic syndromes
Disintegrative psychoses

17.3 SUMMARY: KEY POINTS

• Mental retardation (learning disability) is defined as IQ below 70, with functional impairments in several areas and a childhood onset. Affects 2% of the population.

• Psychiatric and behavioural problems are common, especially in those who also have epilepsy.

• Severe mental retardation is usually caused by genetic or chromosomal abnormalities (e.g. Down's syndrome, fragile X). Mild retardation is often idiopathic and multifactorial.

• Mental retardation is rarely treatable. Management is aimed at maximizing potential and quality of life, and at treating concurrent psychiatric problems. Most people with learning disability live in the community.

CHAPTER 18

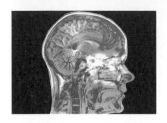

Psychiatry in Non-Psychiatric Settings

The most important message of this book is that psychiatry is part of medicine — there is nothing unique about psychiatric patients or psychiatric disorders when compared to other patients with other illnesses. We have also emphasized that the conventional view of psychiatry, gained from inpatient attachments and some textbooks, shows the specialist tip of the iceberg — most psychiatric disorder presents to, and is dealt with by, GPs and other non-psychiatrists. This chapter extends these themes by describing psychiatric disorder as it is encountered in non-psychiatric settings. It emphasizes that:

• Psychiatric disorders are common in the population and in all areas of medical practice.

• Bodily symptoms are often the presenting feature of psychiatric disorder.

• Psychiatric disorders frequently complicate medical illnesses.

18.1 Epidemiology of psychiatric disorder in non-psychiatric settings

18.1.1 In the population

About 20% of the adult population have a psychiatric disorder at any one time. Neuroses and substance misuse account for most of this morbidity (Table 18.1).

• These are UK data. There are similar American figures.

• Psychiatric morbidity is strongly associated with social deprivation. Rates are two-fold higher in low than high socioeconomic classes, and in urban than rural areas.

• The neuroses are twice as common in women as men; the reverse is true for substance dependence.

• The prevalence for personality disorder, childhood disorders and mental retardation are covered in Chapters 15, 16 and 17, respectively.

Establishing the prevalence of psychiatric disorder

Prevalence data of the kind in Table 18.1 have many limitations, which can lead to misleading (and incompatible) numbers being bandied about:

• Various criteria (e.g. of severity) and diagnostic categories have been used. These especially affect classification of mild neurosis and depression (p. 96), and somatoform disorders (for which there are no good data, though physical symptoms such as fatigue are undoubtedly very common).

• Many cases of neurosis are self-limiting. So the prevalence rates comprise a changing population of people who are transiently and recurrently 'ill'. Other disorders are more often chronic and therefore less sensitive to this effect.

• There is considerable comorbidity. For example, the group of people with neurosis

Table 18.1 Approximate population prevalence of psychiatric disorder.

Disorder	Prevalence (%)
Mixed anxiety–depression	8
Alcohol dependence	5
Generalized anxiety disorder	3
Specific anxiety disorders	3
Depressive disorder	2
Drug dependence	2
Dementia	1
Eating disorders	< 1
Psychosis	0.4

Table 18.2 Adult psychiatric disorders on a typical GP's list.

Number of cases	Disorder
150	Mixed anxiety–depression
100	Alcohol dependence
50	Generalized anxiety disorder
50	Other neuroses (mainly panic and phobic anxiety)
40	Depressive disorder
25	Dementia
10	Psychosis
10	Eating disorders
250	Personality disorder

overlaps with the alcohol dependent and with the personality disordered. This reflects the fact that psychiatric problems are concentrated in a subgroup of the population.

18.1.2 In primary care

How do these population figures apply in primary care? A GP with 2500 people on her list will have roughly the numbers of cases shown in Table 18.2. These figures give an idea of the extent of psychiatric morbidity in the community — and underlie statements such as: 'Half of all GP consultations are for psychiatric problems'. On the other hand, many of the individuals in Table 18.2 will never present with their disorder. The difference between the population prevalence and the number who seek medical help is the first step on the pyramid whose peak is the small and unrepresentative group of psychiatric inpatients (Fig. 18.1).

Psychiatry as seen from general practice

Since psychiatrists and GPs see a different profile of psychiatric disorders, the two groups may have differing views about mental health problems and priorities. For example, a GP may wish to allocate resources to patients with neurotic disorders — who fill her surgeries — whereas her local psychiatrist will probably argue that rarer but more severe disorders take priority.

• The difference in perspective is exemplified by schizophrenia, which is common in specialist psychiatry but not in primary care — a GP only sees a new case every 2 years, and most are then looked after by community mental health teams.

To improve co-ordination between primary care and psychiatric services, several recommendations have been made:
• Psychiatric sector boundaries should reflect GP boundaries.
• Psychiatric and GP training should be closely linked.
• There should be keeping of joint case records.
• GPs and psychiatrists should give consistent information and opinions.
• Responsibility for overall medical care should be held by the GP.
• Local practice guidelines for management should be developed.

18.1.3 In the general hospital

Above and beyond their baseline population prevalence (Table 18.1), particular psychiatric disorders are over-represented in hospital settings.

Casualty departments

Deliberate self-harm is the major psychiatric problem in casualty departments. Although only a minority of cases have persistent psychi-

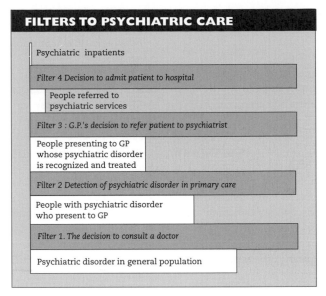

Fig. 18.1 Psychiatric disorders in different settings — the filters to care. Not everyone with a psychiatric disorder presents to their doctor. The decision whether to do so — the first filter — depends on several factors: e.g. awareness that the symptoms may signify psychiatric disorder, the severity of the symptoms, choosing to see a practitioner of alternative medicine, stigma, etc. Of those who do see a doctor, the psychiatric disorder is recognized and treated in about half. This filter to treatment is determined by the issues of recognition and assessment outlined in this chapter and in Chapters 1, 2 and 7. About 10% of patients are referred to psychiatric services; this filter depends on the nature of the disorder, the characteristics of the particular doctor and patient, and the availability of resources. Finally, a tiny minority at some stage have a psychiatric admission. This last filter is based mainly upon the diagnosis (especially psychosis and severe depression), but also on the risk of harm (Chapter 4) and the availability of psychiatric beds and alternative treatment options (Chapter 8).

atric disorders, many have stress and adjustment reactions and some have personality disorders (p. 37). Intoxication and delirium related to alcohol and drugs are also common, particularly in inner cities and in accident victims.

• Some patients with somatoform disorders and a few with factitious disorders (p. 174) are frequent attenders in casualty.

Medical and surgical outpatient clinics

Amongst patients attending medical and surgical outpatient clinics, about a third have physical symptoms which are unexplained — *functional somatic syndromes* (p. 173). Many of them have a psychiatric disorder. Even those who do have a diagnosed disease may well have an accompanying psychiatric disorder — notably depressive and anxiety disorders, adjustment disorder or alcohol misuse.

• In both these groups, adequate recognition and treatment of their psychiatric disorder should be an integral part of management, since it has been shown to improve outcome.

Medical and surgical wards

About 20% of inpatients have a coexisting depressive or anxiety disorder and 10% have a significant alcohol misuse problem. Many elderly inpatients have an episode of delirium (p. 132).

• Some patients with severe somatoform

disorder get admitted and even undergo surgery before the diagnosis is made.

18.2 Presentations of psychiatric disorder in non-psychiatric settings

The recognition of psychiatric disorder in medical settings is not straightforward because it often does not present with the sort of symptoms (e.g. low mood, bingeing) immediately associated with a psychiatric diagnosis. Instead, the presentation may be:

• with medical complaints, either bodily symptoms (e.g. constipation) or hypochondriacal worries;

Fig. 18.2 Psychiatric diagnoses in people with unexplained medical complaints.

• a behavioural problem, such as deliberate self-harm; or
• as the onset or exacerbation of symptoms in the physically ill.

18.2.1 Psychiatric disorder and medical complaints

We have emphasized above and on p. 102 that many patients have persistent symptoms or health anxieties which are medically unexplained. The psychiatric approach to this deceptively large group of patients is summarized in Fig. 18.2.

• The relationship between symptoms, health beliefs and psychiatric disorder is conceptually messy and has led to a large assortment of diagnostic labels. Figure 18.2 is a simplified scheme.

Bodily symptoms due to depressive and anxiety disorders
Depression produces a wide range of bodily

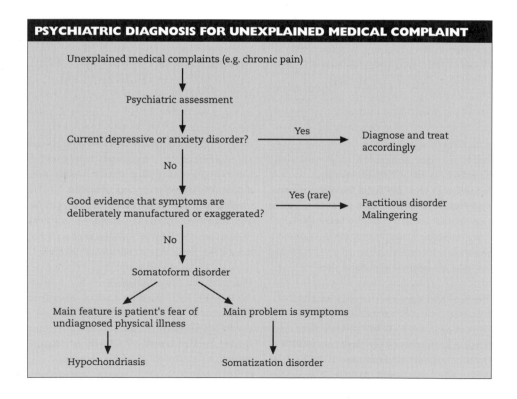

symptoms and signs (p. 84). As a result, a depressed person may be seen in any medical specialty. Similarly, anxiety produces the bodily symptoms of autonomic arousal, including palpitations, breathlessness and paraesthesiae (p. 98); any of these symptoms may be misdiagnosed as evidence of a medical disorder.

Ms M went to her doctor because of abdominal pain. She was upset, but both she and the doctor saw her distress as being a result of the pain. An urgent laparotomy was performed and a normal appendix removed. Only after she took an overdose the following month was a further history taken which revealed that she had been having problems with her mother and had developed symptoms of depressive disorder (low mood, anhedonia and poor sleep) prior to the pain starting. She was given an antidepressant and helped to tackle the family conflict.

So, in any patient who presents with bodily symptoms not clearly explicable by a medical diagnosis, consider the possibility that they have a depressive or anxiety disorder. This process involves both the appropriate investigations to exclude physical disease and the need to seek positive evidence for the presence of depression or anxiety.
• The converse situation — medical disorders producing anxiety and depression — though much rarer, must not be overlooked either (p. 133).

Functional somatic syndromes
The umbrella term *functional somatic syndromes* describes patients who have persistent bodily unexplained symptoms or the belief that they have a serious undiagnosed medical disease (Table 18.3).
• *Functional illness, functional overlay* and other more pejorative labels are used in some circles.
  A large proportion (> 50%) of patients with a functional somatic syndrome satisfy criteria for depressive or anxiety disorder. Clearly if the right questions are not asked, this will not be diagnosed or treated, and the person may

Table 18.3 Common functional somatic syndromes.

Medically unexplained pain syndromes
Non-cardiac chest pain
Facial pain
Pelvic pain
Back pain
Irritable bowel syndrome
Muscular pain and fibromyalgia
Medically unexplained chronic fatigue
Chronic fatigue syndrome

continue to be investigated unnecessarily. Of the patients with a functional somatic syndrome who do *not* have a depressive or anxiety disorder, most have somatization disorder (p. 103).
• Given the prevalence of functional somatic syndromes it is not feasible for all to be seen by psychiatrists. Rather, psychiatric assessment and appropriate treatment should be incorporated into their medical care. Discussion of difficult cases with a liaison psychiatrist may be helpful.

Mr H has attended a gastroenterology clinic intermittently for years with abdominal discomfort and flatulence. No abnormalities have been found despite investigations throughout the length of his gastrointestinal tract. Antispasmodics, laxatives and antiulcer drugs have had no sustained effects. A new junior doctor reviews his case and sees a connection between stresses and the exacerbation of abdominal as well as anxiety symptoms. Mr H is unwilling to countenance a psychological basis for his problems but agrees to see a liaison psychiatrist attached to the clinic. Mr H starts problem-solving therapy and attends a stress management class. His irritable bowel syndrome improves and he agrees (for the first time) that further medical interventions are not necessary.

Factitious disorders and malingering
To add to the complexity there are a few patients who markedly elaborate or make up their symptoms.

• The intentional simulation of symptoms or signs constitutes *factitious disorder* or *malingering*. For example, someone may inject themselves with insulin to produce hypoglycaemia, or collapse and claim they have chest pain. If such behaviour is for obvious gain or fraudulent purposes (e.g. to avoid legal proceedings) it is *malingering*, if its cause is not overt (perhaps it is aimed at receiving the benefits of the sick role; p. 52) it is *factitious disorder*.

• *Munchausen's syndrome* describes people with severe factitious disorder who travel from one hospital to another.

• Some patients simulate psychiatric rather than physical disorder.

• If there is suspicion that symptoms are being manufactured, discrete but determined efforts to verify the person's history should be made. Once a factitious disorder has been confirmed, the patient should be gently confronted with the evidence. However sympathetically the patient is handled, a common response is verbal abuse and self-discharge.

• People with factitious disorder make doctors feel angry and manipulated — most of us have been 'fooled' by a patient with Munchausen's syndrome. These feelings must not spill over to the much larger group of patients who have unexplained medical problems, but in whom there is no evidence for simulation or exaggeration.

18.2.2 Psychiatric disorder presenting with behavioural disturbance

Some psychiatric disorders present because of behaviour which is sufficiently strange, dangerous or otherwise out-of-keeping to bring the person to medical attention one way or another. For example:

• An old lady shouting at imaginary persecutors in casualty.

• A student curled up on her bed hugging her pillow, mute.

• A woman in your GP surgery threatening to cut her wrists or burn her boyfriend's house down.

• A man with no psychiatric history brought in having tried to hang himself.

• A threatening man in the police station having just beaten up his wife.

The diagnosis in these cases proves to be, respectively: delirium; acute stress reaction; personality disorder; psychotic depression; and no psychiatric diagnosis.

• The cases illustrate that any psychiatric disorder can present with a behavioural change, and that a proper assessment is essential. The final example makes the equally important point that people also behave badly for no psychiatric reason at all, and that mental state as well as behaviour must be taken into account when diagnosing psychiatric disorder.

18.2.3 Psychiatric disorder in the medically ill

Many patients with medical disease *also* have psychiatric disorder — the two occur together more often than by chance. Chapter 13 covered the situations where a medical illness produces psychiatric symptoms as part of its pathophysiology. However, there are additional reasons why medical and psychiatric disorder frequently coexist:

• Psychiatric symptoms may be a response to the diagnosis or limitations of a physical disease. For example, depression associated with cancer or sexual dysfunction after myocardial infarction.

• Psychiatric disorder may cause medical illness. For example, osteoporosis in anorexia nervosa.

• There may be a shared cause, such as a major life event precipitating both a stroke and depression.

The coexistence of psychiatric disorder and medical disorder is clinically important because:

• it magnifies suffering and disability;

• it increases mortality in people with heart disease, cancer and stroke; and

• it prolongs medical care and increases overall health costs.

18.3 Management of psychiatric disorder in non-psychiatric settings

There are three main aspects of good management of psychiatric disorder in non-specialist settings. These illustrate the knowledge, skills and attitudes which all doctors should have (p. 2):
• to be able to recognize it;
• to be able to treat it appropriately; and
• to know how and when to refer to specialist psychiatric services.

18.3.1 Recognition

The diagnosis of psychiatric disorder in non-psychiatric settings is often missed. This error may be due to the doctor, the patient or the circumstances (Table 18.4). Doctors are better at the detection and assessment of psychiatric disorder if they:
• realize that bodily complaints are not always due to medical disorders;
• always do a brief psychiatric assessment — this is feasible within any normal time constraint (p. 15);
• identify the patient's worries and concerns;

Table 18.4 Reasons psychiatric diagnoses are missed.

Doctor
Failure to consider the possibility
Failure to elicit psychiatric symptoms — through lack of effort or skill
Patient
Emphasis on bodily complaints
Hides emotional distress and psychosocial stresses
Circumstances
Lack of time
Lack of privacy
Clinic geared toward detection of medical disease

• correct false assumptions about the nature of symptoms and diseases; and
• encourage the expression of emotions and problems.

18.3.2 Treatment

The crucial point is that treatment follows the same principles as it does in specialist psychiatric settings.
• All doctors should be able to provide an appropriate explanation of the disorder to the patient and give advice. Some will use simple psychological therapies (p. 71), others will have staff (e.g. general practice counsellors) who can do so.
• All doctors should be confident to prescribe antidepressants — knowing the indications, practicalities and side-effects (p. 58).

18.3.3 Referral to specialist psychiatric services

An important minority of patients require referral to psychiatric services. The main indications for referral are:
• request for second opinion;
• failure of first-line management;
• need for admission;
• need for specialist treatment, such as ECT;
• suicide risk;
• psychosis;
• substance dependency; and
• need for compulsory treatment.

From primary care, referrals will usually be made to the local general psychiatric services, unless the problem falls into the remit of one of the subspecialties (p. 77). From general hospitals it is more likely to be to the hospital liaison psychiatry service (p. 78).
• Referrals, other than exceptional emergencies, should only be made after the doctor has (a) completed a basic assessment and (b) explained and agreed the referral with the patient.
• Following referral, good communication between all the agencies involved is essential (p. 46).

18.4 SUMMARY: KEY POINTS

- Patients with psychiatric disorders are not only encountered in psychiatry. Patients with neurotic symptoms, depression and anxiety disorders are very common in general practice and general hospitals. In these settings they often present with bodily symptoms.
- Physical illness is frequently accompanied by psychiatric disorder, the presence of which is associated with worse outcomes.
- Psychiatric disorder in both of these non-psychiatric settings can and should be treated in the usual fashion.

- All doctors must be:
  alert to the possibility of psychiatric disorder in their patients;
  aware that psychiatric disorder often presents with bodily symptoms;
  aware of the prevalence of psychiatric disorder in the medically ill;
  able to screen for psychiatric disorder;
  able to use simple psychological treatments;
  able to use antidepressants; and
  aware when and how to refer to psychiatric services.

APPENDIX

Keeping up-to-date and evidence-based

Textbooks and articles can be biased and rapidly outdated. To keep up to date with advances in psychiatry we recommend a textbook of evidence-based medicine (EBM) to hone your EBM skills and knowledge (e.g. *Evidence-based Medicine. How to practice and teach EBM* by Sackett, Richardson, Rosenberg and Haynes. Churchill Livingstone, 1997).

bases is to ask the right question and choose the right key words — see Chapter 2 in the book mentioned above.
- If no RCT is found, search for nonrandomized trials, practice guidelines, or the latest opinion of respected authorities. You may even take note of the opinions expressed in this book . . .

Finding the evidence

To get the best-available answer to therapeutic questions, first search the sources of systematic reviews and other high quality information:
- *Cochrane Library* on CD-ROM, updated quarterly and available in most hospital libraries. It includes the *Cochrane Database of Systematic Reviews* and the *Database of Abstracts of Reviews of Effectiveness*.
- *Best Evidence* — annual CD-ROM compilation of Evidence Based Medicine and ACP Journal Club.
- *Evidence-based Mental Health* — new journal from BMJ Publishing Group. As its editor, JRG admits a vested interest!

If none of these provide an answer, use a database such as MEDLINE, available via terminals in many medical libraries, to search for appropriate randomized controlled trials (RCTs). The secret to searching these data-

Psychiatry on the Net

There are many internet web sites relevant to psychiatry. A useful starting point is the Centre for Evidence–Based Mental Health Website at **http://www.psychiatry.ox.ac. uk/cebmh.html**. This is well linked to:
- Evidence-based medicine resources
- Royal College of Psychiatrists
- Mental Health Act guidelines
- Users' guides
- Psychiatry journals on-line.

There are also sites providing access to resources also available in other forms, such as, MEDLINE, Cochrane Library, biomedical journals, etc.
- Although there is a vast amount of information elsewhere on the web, there are no quality controls and the information is hard to search systematically. Use with caution.

Further Reading

For general reading, the best large textbooks are the *Oxford Textbook of Psychiatry* (3rd edition, 1995, Oxford University Press) and the *Companion to Psychiatric Studies* (6th edition, 1998, Churchill Livingstone).

Chapter 1

Lieberman, J.A. & Rush, J.A. (1996) Redefining the role of psychiatry in medicine. *Am J Psychiatry*, **153**, 1388–1397.

Andreasen, N.C. (1997) What is psychiatry? *Am J Psychiatry*, **154**, 591–593.

Core psychiatry for tomorrow's doctors (1997) *Psychiatr Bull*, **21**, 522–524.

Geddes, J.R. & Harrison, P.J. (1997) Evidence-based psychiatry. Closing the gap between research and practice. *Br J Psychiatry*, **171**, 220–225.

Chapters 2 and 3

Kopelman, M.D. (1994) Structured psychiatric interview. *Br J Hosp Med*, **52**, 93–98 and 277–281.

Davies, T. (1997) Mental health assessment. *BMJ* **314**, 1536–1539.

Chapter 4

Maden, A. (1996) Risk assessment in psychiatry. *Br J Hosp Med*, **56**, 78–82.

Atakan, Z. & Davies, T. (1997) Mental health emergencies. *BMJ*, **314**, 1740–1742.

Hirschfeld, R.M.A. & Russell, J.M. (1997) Assessment and treatment of suicidal patients. *N Engl J Med*, **337**, 910–915.

Harris, E.C. & Barraclough, B. (1997) Suicide as an outcome for mental disorders. A meta-analysis. *Br J Psychiatry*, **170**, 205–228.

Chapter 5

Kendell, R.E. (1975) *The Role of Diagnosis in Psychiatry*. Oxford, Blackwell Scientific Publications

Sharpe, M. (1990) The use of graphical life charts in psychiatry. *Br J Hosp Med*, **44**, 44–47.

Hatcher, S. (1995) Decision analysis in psychiatry. *Br J Psychiatry*, **166**, 184–190.

Chapter 6

Lazare, A. (1973) Hidden conceptual models in psychiatry. *N Engl J Med*, **288**, 345–351.

Cawley, R.H. (1993) Psychiatry is more than a science. *Br J Psychiatry*, **162**, 154–160.

Gelder, M.G. (1996) Biological psychiatry in perspective. *Br Med Bull*, **52**, 401–407.

Plomin, R., Owen, M.J. & McGuffin, P. (1994) The genetic basis of complex human behaviours. *Science*, **264**, 1733–1739.

Chapter 7

Prescribing for the psychiatric patient in the nonspecialist setting (1996) *Prescribers J*, **36**, 181–228.

Andrews, G. (1993) The essential psychotherapies. *Br J Psychiatry*, **162**, 447–451.

Tillett, R. (1996) Psychotherapy assessment and treatment selection. *Br J Psychiatry*, **168**, 10–15.

Enright, S.J. (1997) Cognitive behaviour therapy — clinical applications. *BMJ*, **314**, 1811–1816.

Chapter 8

White, K., Roy, D. & Hamilton, I. (1997) Community mental health services. *BMJ*, **314**, 1817–1820.

Burns, T. (1997) Case management, care management and care programming. *Br J Psychiatry*, **170**, 393–395.

Weich, S. (1997) Prevention of the common mental disorders, a public health perspective. *Psychol Med*, **27**, 757–764.

Chapter 9

Kendler, K.S., Kessler, R.C., Neale, M.C., Heath A.C. & Eaves, L. (1993) The prediction of depression in women: toward an integrated etiologic model. *Am J Psychiatry*, **150**, 1139–1148.

Piccinelli, M. & Wilkinson, G. (1994) Outcome of depression in psychiatric settings. *Br J Psychiatry*, **164**, 297–304.

Scott, J. (1995) Psychological treatments for

depression. An update. *Br J Psychiatry*, **167**, 289–292.

Harris, T.O. & Brown, G.W. (1996) Social causes of depression. *Curr Opin Psychiatry*, **9**, 3–10.

Hale, A.S. (1997) Depression. *BMJ*, **315**, 43–46.

Chapter 10

Gelder, M.G. (1986) Neurosis, another tough old word. *BMJ*, **292**, 972–973.

Hale, A.S. (1996) Anxiety. *BMJ*, **314**, 1886–1889.

Lloyd, K.R., Jenkins, R. & Mann, A. (1996) Long-term outcome of patients with neurotic illness in general practice. *BMJ*, **313**, 26–25.

Mayou, R. & Sharpe, M. (1997) Medically unexplained physical symptoms. *BMJ*, **315**, 561–562.

Chapter 11

Sharp, C.W. & Freeman, C.P.L. (1993) The medical complications of anorexia nervosa. *Br J Psychiatry* **162**, 452–462.

Fairburn, C. (1996) Eating disorders. In *Oxford Textbook of Medicine* (eds D.J. Weatherall, J.G.C. Ledingham & D.A. Warrell), 3rd edn, pp. 4212–4217. OUP, Oxford.

Ashton, C.H. (1997) Management of insomnia. *Prescribers Journal*, **37**, 1–10.

Margison, F.R. (1997) Abnormalities of sexual function and interest, origins and interventions. *Curr Opin Psychiatry*, **10**, 127–131.

Chapter 12

Andreasen, N.C. (1995) Symptoms, signs and diagnosis of schizophrenia. *Lancet*, **346**, 477–481.

Kane, J.M. & McGlashan, T.H. (1995) Treatment of schizophrenia. *Lancet*, **346**, 820–825.

Harrison, P.J. (1997) Schizophrenia, a neurodevelopmental disorder? *Curr Opin Neurobiol*, **7**, 285–289.

Tsuang, M.T. & Faraone, S.V. (1997) *Schizophrenia — The Facts*, 2nd edn. OUP, Oxford.

Chapter 13

Crimlisk, H. & Taylor, M. (1996) How to cope with a neuropsychiatric case. *Br J Hosp Med*, **56**, 103–107.

Trzepacz, P.T. (1996) Delirium. Advances in diagnosis, pathophysiology and treatment. *Psychiatr Clin N Am*, **19**, 429–438.

Small, G.W., Rabins, P.V. *et al.* (1997) Diagnosis and treatment of Alzheimer disease and related disorders. *JAMA*, **278**, 1363–1371.

Harrison, P.J. (1997) BSE and human prion disease. *Br J Psychiatry*, **170**, 298–300.

Lishman, W.A. (1997) *Organic Psychiatry*, 3rd edn. Blackwell Science, Oxford.

Chapter 14

Nutt, D.J. (1996) Addiction, brain mechanisms and their treatment implications. *Lancet*, **347**, 31–36.

Hall, W. & Zador, D. (1997) The alcohol withdrawal syndrome. *Lancet*, **349**, 1897–1900.

Hall, W. & Farrell, M. (1997) Comorbidity of mental disorders with substance misuse. *Br J Psychiatry*, **171**, 4–5.

Schuckit, M.A. (1997) Substance use disorders. *BMJ*, **314**, 1605–1608.

Chapter 15

Tyrer, P., Casey, P. & Ferguson, B. (1991) Personality disorder in perspective. *Br J Psychiatry*, **159**, 463–471.

Stone, M. (1993) Longterm outcome in personality disorders. *Br J Psychiatry*, **162**, 299–313.

Dolan, M. (1994) Psychopathy — a neurobiological perspective. *Br J Psychiatry*, **165**, 151–159.

Marlowe, M. & Sugarman, P. (1997) Disorders of personality. *BMJ*, **315**, 176–179.

Chapter 16

Bailey, A.J. (1993) The biology of autism. *Psychol Med* **23**, 7–12.

Kaplan, C.A. & Hussain, S. (1995) Use of drugs in child and adolescent psychiatry. *Br J Psychiatry*, **166**, 291–298.

Swanson, J.M., Sergeant, J.A., Taylor, E., Sonuga-Barke, E., Jensen, P.S. & Cantwell, D.P. (1998) Attention-deficit hyperactivity disorder and hyperkinetic disorder. *Lancet*, **351**, 429–433.

Spender, Q. & Scott, S. (1996) Conduct disorder. *Curr Opin Psychiatry*, **9**, 273–277.

Hilton, M.R. & Mezey, G. (1996) Victims and perpetrators of child sexual abuse. *Br J Psychiatry*, **169**, 408–415.

Chapter 17

Turk, J. (1992) The fragile-X syndrome. On the way to a behavioural phenotype. *Br J Psychiatry*, **160**, 24–35.

King, B.H., DeAntonio, C., McCracken, J.T., Forness, S.R. & Ackerland, V. (1994) Psychiatric consultation in severe and profound mental retardation. *Am J Psychiatry*, **151**, 1802–1808.

Flint, J. & Wilkie, A.O.M. (1996) The genetics of mental retardation. *Br Med Bull*, **52**, 453–464.

Chapter 18

Paykel, E.S. & Priest, R.G. (1992) Recognition and

management of depression in general practice, consensus statement. *BMJ*, **305**, 1198–1202.

Mayou, R.A. & Sharpe, M. (1995) Psychiatric illness associated with physical disease. *Baillières Clin Psychiatry*, **1**, 201–224.

Craig, T.K. & Boardman, A.P. (1997) Common mental health problems in primary care. *BMJ*, **314**, 1609–1612.

Jenkins, R., Lewis, G., Bebbington, P., Brugha, T., Farrell, M., Grills, B. & Meltzer, H. (1997) The National Psychiatric Morbidity Surveys of Great Britain – initial findings from the Household Survey. *Psychol Med*, **27**, 775–789.

Ramirez, A. & House, A. (1997) Common mental health problems in hospital. *BMJ*, **314**, 1679–1681.

Index

Note: page numbers in *italics* refer to figures and tables, those in **bold** main coverage of topics.